What people are saying

THE FATIGUE

GW00721673

To be listened to and believed is the start of a promising future. You have given me some hope. There are a lot of people who really need this book. Lyn – 72 yrs – CFS/ME

I loved this book. I found it really easy to read. The pages are well laid out and it is broken into short, easy-to-read chapters – perfect for pacing. The illustrations are also great! Lydia writes in a gentle, kind, and supportive way. You can tell that she really has worked with many people to come up with such a helpful and realistic book. After so many years of living with this illness, I hadn't expected to learn much from Lydia but I really have. Laura – 35 yrs – CFS/ME

Since 2020, when my family had COVID, my 16-yr-old son and I have both faced the challenge of long COVID and its non-linear path to recovery. One huge aspect has been navigating the fatigue-laden symptoms. The Fatigue Book is full of practical tips to help manage and minimise the ever-present fatigue on the bumpy road of healing. Jeannie – 49 yrs – long COVID

It is clear that Lydia has a deep understanding, of, and empathy for, those with chronic fatigue. Upon beginning the book, I immediately felt seen. As I continued reading I kept saying 'Yes! Yes! Yes!' with every page turn. I felt as though someone finally knew and understood what I've been going through for many years. Lydia's compassion and gentleness are evident throughout the pages of this book, as is her knowledge of this terrible illness and her experience of helping those who suffer from it. Jacqueline – 38 yrs – CFS/ME

Well done for putting this together. I was interested by the description of cognitive energy. I had assumed that resuming a desk-based job would be possible but actually it drained my energy. I also found some phone calls tiring and would sometimes want to get away. The recovery, very much, is one of stages. There is a high degree of self-discipline in this that is covered in the book. In my case, my first stage of recovery was to walk, starting from almost nothing and advancing by measurable amounts on each excursion. In the middle phase there is very much a need to know when to increase and decrease activity. I so utterly agree with the chapter about Pacing. John – 62 yrs – long COVID

What a significant piece of work this is! It is clearly rooted in wisdom and experience, demonstrating comprehensive understanding of the condition. The tone is right; I love the practical, empowering approach, which covers every detail. I wish this had been available to me years ago. I would have no hesitation in recommending it and feel this book will be of great value to many people. Ann – 65 yrs – CFS/ME and stroke

Wow! This is such a rich resource focusing on the separate strands of a person's experience, equipping them with tools to address each one; then Lydia weaves them all together with a strong message of hope that recovery is not only possible but also achievable! The bite-size format, beautiful illustrations and memorable proverbs transform this book into a life-long companion. Liz – 64 yrs – long COVID

Thanks for the push this book has given me. I might have got there anyway, but it certainly was a motivation in getting started. I had COVID-19 and have struggled since to muster the enthusiasm to do very much at all. It would appear that long COVID had set in and I didn't know for how long. The brain fog began to lift very, very gradually but still the thought of actually doing something was not pleasant. Reading was something I had mostly stopped doing. I began to read this book and my initial thought was, 'I'll never be able to get through this', but I stuck at it, albeit very slowly. By the time I got to Tip 4 'Consider your role in getting better', I realised that it was up to me to try to overcome my own inertia. No one else could do it for me. I hope others get the benefit of your obvious experience and knowledge. Ray – 65 yrs – long COVID

Wow! This book spoke directly to me and reassured me right from the start. Having discussed health issues (headaches, poor sleep, digestive issues, brain fog) with my doctor, this is the first time I have ever heard it suggested they could be linked. I have really understood the necessity of practising fatigue management! I honestly think this book is what I've been waiting for without even realising it.
Vivienne – 58 yrs – undiagnosed chronic fatigue and long COVID

THE FATIGUE BOOK

Chronic fatigue syndrome and long COVID fatigue:
Practical tips for recovery

Lydia Rolley Dip COT, MSc

Illustrations by Rachel Alice Leggett

With a Foreword by
Dr Charlotte Merriman

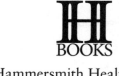

Hammersmith Health Books
London, UK

First published in 2022 by Hammersmith Health Books
– an imprint of Hammersmith Books Limited
4/4A Bloomsbury Square, London WC1A 2RP, UK
www.hammersmithbooks.co.uk

Disclaimer:
This book is designed to provide helpful information on the subjects discussed. It is not meant to be used, nor should it be used, to diagnose or treat any medical condition. For diagnosis or treatment of any medical problem, consult your own physician or healthcare provider. The publisher and author are not responsible for any specific health or allergy needs that may require medical supervision and are not liable for any damages or negative consequences from any treatment, action, application or preparation, to any person reading or following the information in this book. References are provided for informational purposes only and do not constitute endorsement of any websites or other sources. Readers should be aware that the websites listed in this book may change. The information and references included are up to date at the time of writing but given that medical evidence progresses, it may not be up to date at the time of reading.

British Library Cataloguing in Publication Data:
A CIP record of this book is available from the British Library.

Print ISBN 978-1-78161-237-8
Ebook ISBN 978-1-78161-238-5

Commissioning editor: Georgina Bentliff
Designed and typeset by: Madeline Meckiffe
Cover design by: Madeline Meckiffe
Illustrations and cover image by: Rachel Alice Leggett
Index: Dr Laurence Errington
Production: Deborah Wehner of Moatvale Press Ltd
Printed and bound by: TJ Books Ltd, Cornwall, UK

CONTENTS

FOREWORD

I first met Lydia Rolley when I came for interview at the specialist CFS/ME Service in Sheffield. Despite our paths having never crossed before, her warmth and generosity of spirit were evident in that very first and brief meeting. There was something unique and captivating about her compassion and gentleness that intrigued me. I wanted to know her more. Since that time, Lydia has now grown to be one of my greatest inspirations and most adored friends. Throughout the time I had the privilege of working alongside her, prior to her recent retirement, I saw her kind wisdom and compassionate spirit transform the lives of those most in need, time and time again. Her ability to be alongside people with love, hope and gentleness, and without judgement, was uniquely healing.

I hope that in reading this book you will be able to receive a distillation of Lydia's essence in its pages. Certainly, when I read it I can hear her voice and sense the love and wisdom contained within it. I am so proud of her willingness to follow the path of writing this book. I know she was fearful and uncertain at the start, just as you may be at the start of your journey with chronic fatigue now. However, she did not let that fear hold her back, and with courage she repeatedly took the small steps to put to paper all that she had learned in her journey of supporting those with chronic fatigue in her professional life, so that you can benefit from it now.

Lydia's faith is an exceedingly important part of who she is as a person, and what guides her in her life. To those who know her, this faith shines through in all that she says or does. I am not a Christian, and nor do I hold a faith. However, knowing Lydia, and seeing how her faith guides her to make such a difference to people's lives, makes me curious about there being a power higher than ourselves which can heal and guide us in our darkest moments.

When we worked together, Lydia would often talk about people having little hope at the start of their journey with chronic fatigue, and how it is important at that time for us to 'hold the hope for them'. It does not matter in reading this book if you have no faith, or a different faith; all I would encourage you to do is to be open to what she has to offer. If nothing else, maybe you can let Lydia's faith in her God hold you now in your current uncertainty, and as a scientist practitioner I can hold the scientific faith that these methods can and will lead to your recovery, if applied with patience, determination and courage.

I can also endorse the ideas contained within this book from personal experience. Ten years ago, I similarly found myself struggling with debilitating fatigue and a host of troubling and disabling symptoms, which were not explainable by blood tests or investigations. The descriptions written in this book could well have been written about me. Although I worked hard at finding my own way through those health challenges to the better place I now find myself in, I wonder how much shorter my season of ill-health would have been if I'd had access to Lydia's book back then. I cannot help but think what a gift that would have been. And so, let Lydia's hard work in collating these tips and strategies lighten the load for you as you undertake this journey, and let the planting of the seeds begin for your new season of renewed health.

Dr Charlotte Merriman
Senior Clinical Psychologist

To all my past patients
for inspiring me to write.

ABOUT THE AUTHOR

Lydia is a recently retired occupational therapist (DipCOT – Salford College of Occupational Therapy, 1982) and systemic psychotherapist/family therapist (MSc – Leeds University, 2011). Throughout her career she has worked in a variety of mental and physical health NHS settings, including over 15 years as part of a specialist regional chronic fatigue management service.

As well as her NHS career, Lydia worked with her family in Croatia and Bosnia Herzegovina, supporting humanitarian aid causes during the Balkan war in the mid-1990s. Her youngest of four children, Rachel Alice Leggett, was born in Zagreb, Croatia. She is the illustrator of *The Fatigue Book*.

Lydia has her own lived experience of CFS/ME and, when diagnosed many years ago, was given no support or guidance. She rarely talks about her experience, but it has fuelled her desire, over the years, to work collaboratively and enable people in their recovery journey.

Sheffield has been her home for many years. She loves spending time with family and friends and exploring all that Sheffield and the surrounding beautiful countryside have to offer.

ABOUT THE ILLUSTRATOR

Rachel is a talented artist, who uses a wide range of styles and mediums. She has been drawing since she could pick up a pencil.

She obtained her foundation diploma in Art, Design and Media at Chesterfield College (2013), her Theatre Design BA (Hons) degree at Nottingham Trent University (2017) and Creative Graphics for Marketing & Communications (2022).

She is married and currently lives and works in Nottingham.

INTRODUCTION

The morning starts ... or, should I say, the mid-morning starts.

As you lie in bed trying to stay awake, you wonder: 'Is this day going to be any better than yesterday?'

Getting out of bed takes you longer than you anticipated – not through lack of desire though. You wonder why your body feels so heavy all the time. You wander through to the bathroom, feeling unrefreshed after a long but restless night. You question why you couldn't sleep even though you were exhausted.

You decide to wear some simple clothes today. You are not planning on going anywhere. A quick wash will do this morning. Showers used to wake you up and help you feel fresh and ready for the day; now they perhaps leave you wanting to climb back into bed.

You eventually make it to the kitchen, wondering if you can still call this breakfast, as it is now past lunchtime. You certainly don't have the appetite you used to. Your tastes have changed and your previous love for inventive cooking seems a world away.

Currently, you are off work on sick leave. Before this year, you have never taken time off work due to illness. You tried to go back to work but only managed a couple of days and then completely crashed. That was weeks ago, and you are still recovering now. All your other symptoms are exacerbated.

As you are drinking your cup of tea, you feel grateful that no one is at home and there is some quiet. You check your phone; despite reading only a few kind messages, you sense a headache starting. A physical headache – sore eyes, pounding temples, you struggle to concentrate and process what you are reading. Also, a dilemma-type headache. You wonder how to respond to well-meaning friends. They don't have a clue as to how you really are. It is so difficult to put into words or answer the simple but dreaded question of *'How are you?'* You used to be the life and soul of the party but now a message or phone call can leave you wrecked.

You decide to lie on the settee for just five minutes. You know you would feel more comfortable back on your bed, but the stairs leave you breathless and in pain. Before you know it, two hours have passed and you wake, feeling worse than you did before ...

Sounds familiar?

This may not be exactly the same as parts of your story, but the traits are probably similar. Stories like this are repeated thousands of times, up and down the country, and in fact throughout our present-day world. Many stories of chronic fatigue, unheard and unseen. The Office for National Statistics (ONS)[1] estimates that, at the beginning of March 2021, over a million people in the UK had reported symptoms associated with long COVID (also known as post-COVID-19 syndrome or 'long haulers'). By April 2022 this number had risen to 1.7 million people in the UK – 2.7% of the population.[2] More than half of these people reported that their ability to undertake their day-to-day activities had been negatively impacted by their symptoms. Fatigue is the most dominant and widely reported symptom. Long COVID is a relatively new thing, but chronic fatigue is not. Chronic fatigue syndrome/ myalgic encephalomyelitis (CFS/ME) has been around for a long time. Countless people of all ages suffer from this condition, which has often been misunderstood, overlooked and under-resourced. Despite some of the reported differences between these two conditions and the many unknowns of long COVID, there is significant overlap. Both are relapsing and remitting conditions that present with fluctuating, ongoing, profound and debilitating fatigue – chronic fatigue.

This book addresses chronic fatigue. It outlines proven fatigue management tips and is suitable for people of all ages affected by either long COVID or CFS/ME. Whether you are at the start of your recovery journey or have been doing this for some time now, there are useful tips within these pages. It uses a self-management approach in applying the principles of Pacing and Activity Management as recommended by NICE guidelines[3, 4] for both conditions, many of which are being used in the recently set-up long COVID clinics, or 'hubs', to treat fatigue.

This book is also a rich resource for professionals and family members wanting to learn how they can better support patients and family members affected by chronic fatigue.

I worked for the final 15 years of my NHS career in fatigue management, in a regional specialist service for CFS/ME. My planned retirement as an Occupational Therapist and Family Therapist/Systemic Psychotherapist came in August 2020, in the middle of the pandemic. I have worked with a wide range of conditions, both in physical and mental health, but nothing has stretched or challenged me as much as chronic fatigue.

I have had the enormous privilege of working with committed, creative and hard-working colleagues. We all wanted to serve our patients well and help discover the solutions together with them. Within this collaborative patient-led approach, we witnessed numerous adults, families, young people and children affected by chronic fatigue, turn their lives around and take steps of recovery towards healthier, freer lives.

I wanted to make the therapy sessions useful and not waste anyone's precious time, especially when energy was so low, in order to co-create some clarity, reflection, solutions and direction. I wanted to move forwards in small ways with patients, to their desired outcome and preferred future, in the midst of the dominating fatigue. This is also my desire in writing this book.

It is my simple contribution to addressing the ever-increasing need in our current-day world of chronic fatigue.

HOW TO USE THIS BOOK

- **Patiently** – You cannot rush fatigue management. It takes time and steady perseverance. Don't read it from cover to cover either: take it slowly. Pace yourself and be kind to yourself.

- **Simply** – The tips are written simply and succinctly, and are mostly illustrated. You can just concentrate on one tip at a time. For some of you affected by brain fog, reading, concentration, retaining and processing information may be limited.

> The main nugget from each tip has been highlighted, as this paragraph is. This allows you to focus just on that section, with the option to read more if capacity and desire permit.

- **Individually or collectively** – This book is suitable for working through on your own or you can follow the Pacing Group Guidelines (Appendix 3) to complete with one or two others.

- **Willingly** – Throughout the tips, there are suggestions of how to apply the principles outlined. If you feel comfortable, be willing to have a go and try putting the tips into practice.

- **Hopefully** – These tips have all worked in other people's lives. Each tip brings somebody to mind and was no doubt discussed together in a therapy session. I have seen each tip bring progress and the desired change to someone's life. Commencing a rehabilitation journey, like this one, can feel somewhat overwhelming and, at times, hope can be hard to find. We often need others to hope on our behalf until our own hope grows.

STRUCTURE OF THIS BOOK

Each chapter is a topic in itself and can be read in isolation. If we were in therapy sessions together and *Anxiety* or *Sleep* were the most pressing issues for you, that would be our focus. However, understanding *Energy* and applying the details of *Pacing and activity management* do not come easily. People can think they understand these and brush over them, when actually they hold the key to the change you are seeking – better health and more energy.

Change happens when the smallest of steps are done consistently over a long period of time. This book will not change you but your collaboration with it will and can.

At the end of each chapter are three short sections:

- **Food for thought** – This is a quote, a thought or a fact that is related to the topic of the chapter.

- **Pause** – This is a practical exercise or activity to try.

- **Mind, body and soul** – This closes each chapter and is intended to be the most holistic part of the chapter. It is an opportunity to reflect on your thoughts about the topic, how you plan to put it into practice and to maybe consider the spiritual as part of your recovery journey. As human beings, we are mind, body and soul – whole people. Often the spiritual can get neglected until times of crisis. During the pandemic, the fragility of health and life has brought this subject more to the fore for most of us. I am aware of the wide spectrum of beliefs and non-beliefs amongst readers. This is a chance to have a slow-down-stop moment. A chance to reflect on the topic of the chapter and, if you feel comfortable, there is a written prayer from a Christian perspective, inviting God's help in the recovery process.

My desire is that, together with your collaboration, this book will be useful for you in your recovery journey.

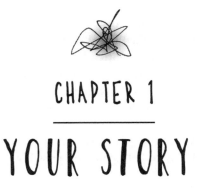

CHAPTER 1

YOUR STORY

To be honest with you, I would much rather sit and hear your story and chat back and forth, rather than for you to be reading this book. Despite having the same diagnosis as other people, everyone has their own story to tell. Yours is no exception and totally unique.

I would be curious to know what your life was like prior to experiencing chronic fatigue and how chronic fatigue has affected your life. I would love to hear about your hopes and desires, your family and friends. Also, about what motivates you, what hobbies or special interests you have. Maybe you would tell me about significant events that have shaped and influenced you, for better or for worse.

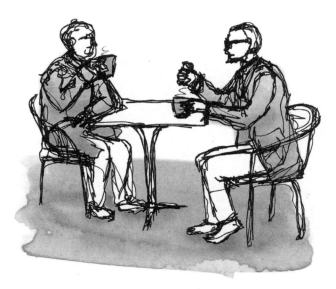

At this point, I would dearly love to place an enormous magnifying glass over your strengths and abilities and any previous stories of hope, resilience and overcoming. These tend to get forgotten or overlooked when faced with such poor health. But they are still a part of who you are. Chronic fatigue, as with a lot of chronic illnesses, is often like a thief that tries to steal those parts of your story by coming along and dominating your life.

I would be interested to know how you became ill and what life was like for you at the time. No doubt, most areas of your life have been turned upside down, and side to side, by this fatigue and you are currently not able to function in ways that you previously could. It would be important to consider what your expectations and hopes are for your recovery journey and what things are likely to help you, and possibly hinder you, in that journey.

> My hope is that by considering *your story* at the start of this book, *you* are put at the centre of this book first and foremost. It is your journey of recovery. I hope that your unique needs are met and that your own self and personality are expressed as you take steps forward in dealing with the fatigue and moving towards the recovery that *you* want.

That which does blossom in the spring will bring forth fruit in the autumn.
British proverb

TIP 1: THIS IS A SEASON IN YOUR LIFE

What you are going through at present is for a season – it is your present reality, but it is not your life. You have a past, a present and a future and are not meant to stay in this season for the rest of your life.

You may have been in this season for quite a while already, or you may have just started experiencing chronic fatigue. Even though I have not met you, I am sure that I can say, with all certainty, that it is not a season you have either wanted or chosen. It is a very real, very painful, very present and very costly season.

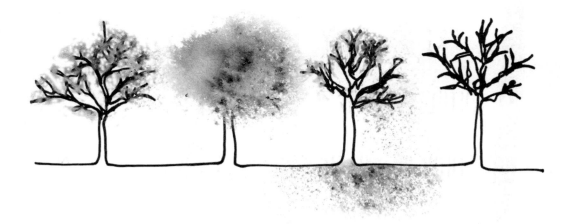

It will not always be like this.
I have seen countless people move through this season.

What we are unable to answer at this point in time is: *'How long will this season last?'* It may well be a much longer season than you want it to be. You will need the gift of patience and hope to travel through it.

As with nature's seasons, some things grow, and some things may end up looking completely different. In autumn, old things fade and in spring, new things come to life. Change takes place. For you, new habits can grow, old habits may go.

It will not always be like this. This season is for now – but not forever.

STRENGTHS

HONE**S**TY

POSI**T**IVITY

HUMOU**R**

FRI**E**NDLY

AUTHE**N**TIC

THOU**G**HTFUL

CURIOSI**T**Y

T**H**INKER

AS**S**ERTIVE

ABILITIES

DR**A**WS

BAKES

WR**I**TES

PI**L**ATES

PA**I**NTS

CRAF**T**S

SW**I**MS

POTT**E**RY

SPORT

TIP 2: REMEMBER YOUR STRENGTHS AND ABILITIES

Chronic illness can be so dominating and confidence-stealing. It can take so much time, attention and focus just to get through a day. Symptoms can scream loudly and be all-consuming. The fatigue can cause you to be unable to fully function and operate as you used to do. Oftentimes, the fatigue masks who you really are, and your strengths hardly get to see the light of day.

It is so easy to forget that your strengths and abilities are still there. They are extraordinary resources that have equipped you to live your life so far. They have given you resilience and hope during previous challenging times in your life. You need to be able to draw upon them for this recovery journey.

Picture the sun during the wintertime. The sun is the same size, strength and brightness every day of the year, but in the winter months it is often hidden. We do not see or experience it as often, but it is still the same sun.

You are still who you are, with all your strengths and abilities – amazing and unique.

Stop now and consider some of your strengths and abilities. It may be useful to get someone else to assist you with this. List at least two of your strengths and abilities and be thankful for each one. Remind yourself often of these. They may not be fully seen and known by others in this season – but you know. They will enable you to reach towards your preferred future.

When the sun is highest it casts the least shadow.
British proverb

TIP 3: NOTE YOUR GENERAL ATTITUDE TO ILLNESS

Prior to the chronic fatigue, what was your general attitude to illness? Were you a 'get on with it' type of person? Maybe you rarely took a day off work and perhaps did not have a lot of compassion for those who did? Or perhaps you were a 'go to bed' type of person when illness came along?

Identifying your general attitude to illness may be obvious and straightforward for you. If not, consider what your parents' attitude to illness was. My parents, for example, held opposite views. One had a 'get on with it' attitude and one had a 'go to bed' attitude. I quickly learnt which parent to go to when I was sick and not wanting to go to school. Another way to highlight your attitude to illness is to consider what advice you would give to another family member or friend if they were ill.

Another attitude to illness that I have encountered has been 'let it take its course', 'what will be, will be' and 'it will get better in time'. This kind of laid-back attitude may be appropriate for certain illnesses, like the flu or a cold, where you have to sit it out and wait for it to go. However, in longer-term health conditions like chronic fatigue, this lack of intervention or intentionality only serves to prolong the condition and promote further deconditioning.

You may hold one of the attitudes above or you may hold some other point of view. Just spend a moment to consider your attitude.

Why is it useful to take note of your general attitude to illness? Rehabilitation from fatigue requires balance. At times, this means doing things that can feel counterintuitive or the opposite way to your natural response. This can feel wrong and awkward at times, but it does work. These attitudes for dealing with various illnesses have served you well in the past and will continue to do so for certain conditions, but, for this recovery journey, the middle ground will probably serve you better.

Good health is a crown worn by the healthy that only the ill can see.
Arabic proverb

TIP 4: CONSIDER YOUR ROLE IN GETTING BETTER

With a lot of illnesses, we go to the doctor to be given a diagnosis and, more importantly, a cure or treatment to fix it and ideally make it go away. With chronic fatigue, most of the treatment is down to self-management. In other words, it is not something that can be done to you but is something you must take on board and do yourself.

If you have long COVID or CFS/ME you may have been fortunate enough to have a multi-disciplinary team assessment. It is important to have a medical assessment to correctly diagnose long COVID or CFS/ME and to identify or rule out any comorbid conditions. You may have been advised that some symptoms require medical monitoring (such as respiratory, neurological or cardiac symptoms). You will need intervention from medical professionals for those conditions. But as far as the chronic fatigue rehabilitation is concerned, the professionals can teach, encourage and support you, but only *you* can put the principles of fatigue management into practice.

I can honestly say that, in all my years of clinical practice, I have seen hundreds of people move towards recovery, but it has required each of them to put fatigue management into practice. I commend every single one of them.

As you start this recovery journey, just take a moment to consider your expectations of other people. Are you expecting professionals to fix you? Or hoping family members will step in? Maybe you need to readjust some of these expectations? Seek out professionals, as well as family and friends, who can be on your support team – those people who will encourage and monitor your progress, reassure and motivate you with the self-management journey ahead.

Only *you* can put the principles of fatigue management into practice.

Teachers open the door, but you must enter by yourself.
Chinese proverb

TIP 5: GETTING BACK TO 'NORMAL'

I don't know about you, but certainly since the start of the COVID-19 pandemic, in 2020, a lot of people have talked about 'getting back to normal'. More recently, we have talked about the 'new normal' because none of us are quite sure what 'normal' looks like anymore. We have all had to be somewhat flexible and hopeful in the midst of uncertainty and restrictions.

In some ways, recovery from chronic fatigue is similar. I have witnessed countless people recover from this, and most have gone on to function well in all areas of their life.

For many of them, however, their new normal is not the same as their old normal, or even the normal they thought they were aiming for. They may now have different perspectives, desires, priorities and outlooks on life. Some have changed life direction, careers and friendship groups.

Those who have done well, in the midst of all the uncertainty, have needed to be flexible in their thinking, yet able still to maintain a hopeful view of their future and recovery.

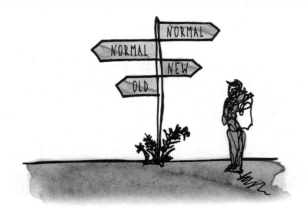

Chameleons change colour to match the earth; earth doesn't change colour to match the chameleons.
Senegalese proverb

TIP 6: BEING UNDERSTOOD

Being misunderstood or not believed, or having to justify and fight one's case, is absolutely exhausting. I have seen this issue alone set people back months in their recovery process. Conversely, I have seen the relief and the accompanying physical exhalation when someone knows that they have been understood.

I am sure that there are many times when you, yourself, do not understand what is going on, so it is challenging for significant others to understand too.

Oftentimes, the fatigue and its effects are unseen. The fatigue tends to keep you hidden. By that, I mean that you can only be seen and known on a 'good' or 'better' day – when you have the energy to meet with others or venture out. This can contribute to people not understanding the whole presentation.

It is unrealistic to expect everyone to understand, because they won't

The whole world is still trying to get its head around COVID-19 and long COVID fatigue. It is encouraging that more clinics and professionals are being trained in awareness of long COVID fatigue and chronic fatigue management. The CFS/ME community has waited years to be better understood.

Find the ones and twos who do understand

For close family and friends, give them information to read for themselves. Choose a time, when you have more energy, to explain to them some of your experiences and what is helpful and what is not.

Think of a one liner

You may get asked questions about your health that you do not want or need to answer. Often this can occur at times when you do not have the energy or desire to continue in a certain conversation. It can be useful to have a planned short response that remains diplomatic but closes the conversation down. An example could be: 'Thanks for your interest but I would rather hear about…'

Avoid battles and conflicts

These will only use up your energy and exacerbate your symptoms. Having to prove to others that you are unwell makes the illness worse. I have worked with patients who ended up changing doctors, schools, colleges, workplaces, friendship groups and social groups. Their recovery journey took a turn for the better after they had settled into less conflictual situations. I am reminded of the phrase 'choose your battles'. Battles are costly for your health. Some you can drop, some you can resolve, some you can delegate and some you maybe have to fight, but be wise.

Just take a moment to consider this topic. Consider who understands your situation the most. Be thankful for them. Is there anything you can do to further people's understanding of your health needs? Are there any battle situations you, or someone on your behalf, needs to change?

There can be no peace without understanding.
African proverb

TIP 7: YOUR ROAD TO RECOVERY

As we do not know exactly how long your journey may take, or how many stops and starts, twists and turns, there may be for you, let us look at the different stages of this journey – the Beginning, Middle and End. Let us consider together some of the characteristics that may occur at each of these stages.

This list is not exhaustive, and I am sure that you may well have characteristics to add to the list. As you read it, consider your journey and all those who have gone before, who are helping to point out the direction of the path to take.

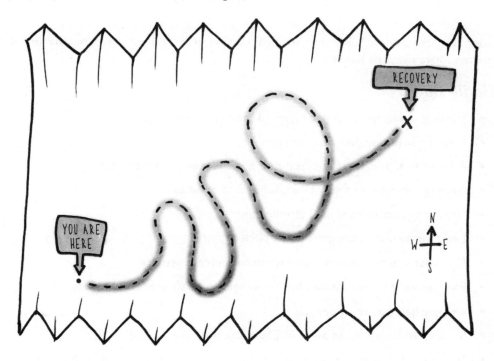

Beginning stage

- Ill and very fatigued – the importance of getting a medical overview and diagnosis
- Searching for answers – trying to make sense of it all

- Looking to authorities to make you better
- Extremes in 'booming and busting'
- Fear and anxiety
- Shock/trauma/confusion of it all
- Hard to see the way forward – time needed for all the dust to settle
- Adjustments/losses
- No longer independent – more dependent
- Acceptance (or not) of the diagnosis and treatment pathway
- Steep learning curve with regard to fatigue management
- Starting to reflect and learn from everyday situations.

During this stage: confusion moves towards clarity, uncertainty moves towards direction, extremes move towards balance.

Middle stage

- Starting to engage with pacing and activity management
- Frequently taking preventative rests
- A lot of trial and error but continuing with fatigue management
- Greater awareness of self, body, limits and abilities
- Gradually becoming skilled at reflecting
- Learning to plan, anticipate and switch activities
- Knowing when to increase and when to decrease activity
- Experiencing some setbacks but these tend to be shorter and less frequent
- Greater balance, less payback
- Starting to re-engage in areas of life in small ways
- Willing to try small steps rather than staying safe, out of fear of getting worse.

During this stage: consistency, balance and small steady steps of progress are hallmarks. Still uncertainty.

End stage

- Continues with all the characteristics of the middle stage
- Pacing and resting are part of life
- Continuing to make steady, small steps of progress
- Boredom and a desire to do more
- Some setbacks from attempting more, but able to turn them around more quickly than before
- Able to function better in all areas of life
- Perhaps adapted or changed some decisions in life
- Knowing how to manage health, independently of professional support
- Able to reflect and learn from the positives and negatives of this season

During this stage: confidence, resilience and stability are hallmarks and dependence moves towards independence. Active acceptance.

As you consider your own road to recovery, write down:

- two to three things that may hinder you or get in the way. What can be done, if anything, about these?
- two to three things that may help you on your way. What can be done, if anything, to facilitate these?

The prudent give thought to their steps.
Book of Proverbs[NIV]

TIP 8: ONE SIZE DOESN'T FIT ALL

I have seen all the tips in this book applied to different individuals' lives and have had the privilege of seeing them work in their recovery journey.

They really do work.

Having said that, each person is unique. How one person presents with fatigue symptoms may be very similar to someone else. However, their recovery journey, both in terms of how long and what is involved, may look somewhat different.

As you read this book and consistently try to put these principles into practice, you will discover what works for you and what does not. This whole journey, though based on evidence, is patient-driven and also one of trial and error.

I encourage you to be willing to give them all a try. You may surprise yourself with which tips work for you.

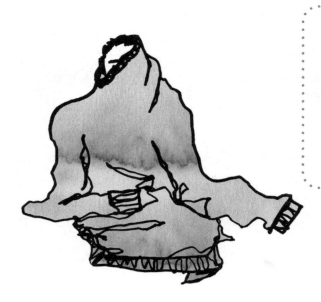

There are many paths to the top of the mountain but the view is always the same.
Chinese proverb

TIP 9: CHOOSE YOUR WORDS WISELY

Our words are powerful. We all know how damaging it is when someone speaks critically against us. Those words sting and stick with us for quite a while. Conversely, words of encouragement can build us up and boost how we are feeling.

> Just take a moment and consider what words you have spoken about yourself, or to yourself, recently? Have you, by any chance, used any of the following types of descriptions, or words?

'Oh, you idiot.'

'I am so stupid.'

'Dumb or what?'

'I am so thick.'

Certainly, in the UK, we tend to use self-criticism a lot more readily than self-praise. It is understandable to get frustrated. You are currently not able to function as you have been able to. The fatigue has done this to you.

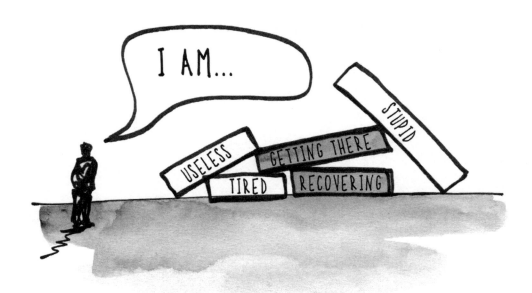

Reframing what you say is a therapeutic way of creating a different language and perspective. 'Oh, you idiot,' reframed could be, 'Oh, I made a mistake, but 10 out of 10 for effort.'

This cannot be done in the heat of the moment. Try taking some time to reflect on things you frequently say and consider an alternative way, which expresses things truthfully but builds you up rather than tears you down.

Be aware of what you say to yourself. Try speaking out loud – words of encouragement to yourself throughout the day – for the small things as well as the large ones.

Be kind to yourself. It's important.

Gracious words are … sweet to the soul
and healing to the bones.
Book of Proverbs^{NIV}

TIP 10: YOUR HOPES AND AIMS ARE CRUCIAL

Your hopes and aims are crucial – I really do mean *crucial*. They are essential for your recovery, as they stir motivation and help you persevere when the going gets tough.

To hope means to anticipate goodness. It implies wanting something to happen for the better and sensing expectation for the future. You tend to align your aims and goals in life with your hopes. An aim is a purpose or intention or a desired outcome.

When chronic illness looms large along with losses, repeated disappointments and difficulties, it can be challenging to hold onto even the smallest amount of hope. Sometimes just the thought of being hopeful, in the midst of that level of disappointment, can feel somewhat incongruent.

At this point, I encourage you to consider your aims. What aims and hopes come to mind as you read this tip? What is your aim in reading this book? What are some of your aims in getting better?

'*I want to be able to …*'

'*I hope that …*'

Write down two or three of your aims and consider what helps you hold onto hope.

A longing fulfilled is sweet to the soul.
Book of Proverbs[NIV]

FOOD FOR THOUGHT

Wisely and slow;
They stumble that run fast.
William Shakespeare[5]

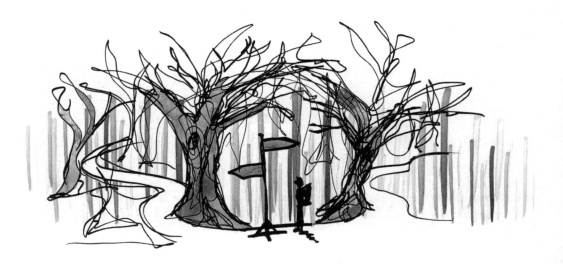

PAUSE: STOPPING

Stop what you are doing.

Move and find a quiet spot.

Turn off all background noises.

Sit and just be still and peaceful for at least 3 minutes.

Nothing more, nothing less.

Practise this often throughout your day.

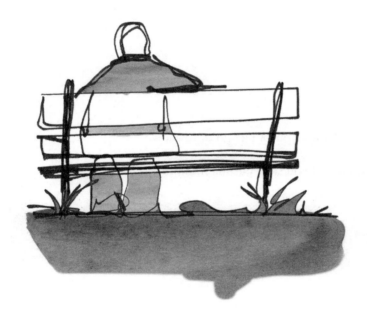

MIND, BODY AND SOUL: YOUR STORY

Mind: What were your thoughts as you read this chapter on Your story?

Other parts of the chapter you can let go of for now.

Body: What actions will you start putting into practice?

Soul: You may want to seek soul help with these changes. As explained in the book's introduction, this section is from my perpective as a Christian, inviting God's help in the recovery process. You may have your own way of seeking soul help, so please do what you feel comfortable with.

Dear God
I ask you for help with my story and my recovery journey.
'You know when I sit and when I rise ... You discern
my going out and my lying down ... I praise you because
I am fearfully and wonderfully made ... How precious to me
are your thoughts, God! How vast is the sum of them!'[NIV]
Thank you God.
Amen ... may it be so.
Based upon Psalm 139[6]

CHAPTER 2

THE FATIGUE

The greater the understanding and awareness you have of the fatigue and its characteristics, the more you can learn to manage it. With time, the better the fatigue is managed, the less it will affect you.

The fatigue is something that has dominated and affected countless lives with detrimental effects. One of my greatest joys is seeing people take steps away from the fatigue, towards freedom, little by little. It is possible and it does work.

I wonder how you would describe the fatigue. I would love to hear. Let us imagine that it is a character, and we are describing it to someone who has no idea who or what fatigue is like. What would you say? How would you describe its characteristics? What does it do? What are its strategies? What are its effects on you and your body? What are its effects on those around you and your relationships?

Let me start by telling you some of the kinds of descriptions of the fatigue that I have heard; some may sound familiar to you. Please consider your own as we go:

- Sometimes the fatigue is too close and dominates every moment of the day and night. Occasionally, it moves further away and lets you enjoy doing something without bothering you quite so much – but then it comes back with a vengeance, and you end up paying heavily for that short reprieve, the next day, and the day after that too. This pay back after activity is also known as post-exertional malaise (PEM).

- Most days you are aware of the fatigue. From the moment you wake up, it makes your body feel heavy and it is hard to get out of bed.

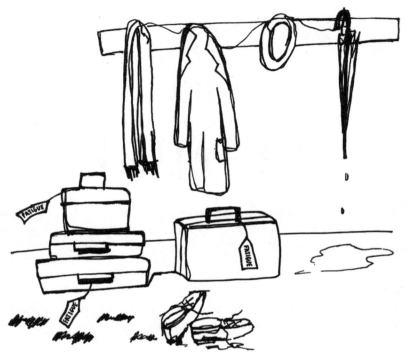

- The fatigue is like an unwelcome guest who has come and stayed in your life and home for too long already. It is constantly there and won't go away by itself.

- Usually, when the fatigue is very present and dominant, it brings its own company and it can all get a bit too much. The company includes other symptoms, like headaches, pain, brain fog, aching muscles and joints, and poor concentration. Usually, the more fatigue there is, the worse all the other symptoms become.

- The fatigue wants you to rest all day and do nothing, but this only causes it to continue.

- Sometimes you want to fight the fatigue by pushing through and keeping going – a kind of mind-over-matter type attitude, trying to do activities that you previously did with ease. Sadly, this also only causes the fatigue to continue.

- The fatigue makes everyday activities difficult.

- At times, the fatigue can be invisible to other people, but you are aware of it all the time.

This chapter looks at ways to understand the fatigue and its boom and bust nature. It will equip you with some starter tips in learning how to manage the fatigue.

TIP 11: BECOME AN EXPERT ON THE FATIGUE

When patients came to see me for the first time, I often told them that I was not an expert on their body, their circumstances or their experience of the fatigue. They were the experts, not me.

What I did bring to the table was some expertise in fatigue management. This had been gleaned over many years as a therapist, witnessing other people's journeys with fatigue and recovery from it.

Therapy consisted of collaborating with patients to use our joint expertise to shed light and co-create solutions and ways forward.

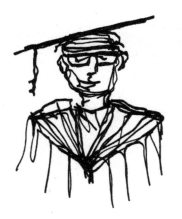

The patients soon became the experts in their fatigue management, often through trial and error and learning from recent experiences. This equipped them to manage the fatigue, not letting it dominate their lives, and move towards their goals and aspirations.

The more that you can manage the fatigue, the less it will manage you.

The heart of the discerning acquires knowledge.
Book of Proverbs[NIV]

TIP 12: IF YOU DON'T WANT THE FATIGUE, DON'T CALL IT YOURS

For some reason, we often use personalised language to refer to chronic illnesses:

- 'My fatigue'
- 'My pain'
- 'My stress'
- 'My anxiety'

Instead of saying, 'My fatigue', start saying, 'The fatigue'.

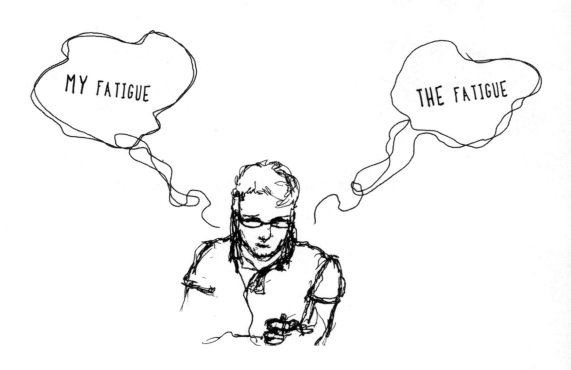

This may sound like splitting hairs but I have seen many patients make this small change in their language and, over time, it has changed their perspective. It does take practice.

> By externalising your language to describe the chronic fatigue, it can create some distance between you and the fatigue. This helps you consider how it is affecting you and what your relationship to it is at that point in time. It can give you a sense of control.

For example:

- 'I went for a short walk and the fatigue just came on me suddenly.'
- 'The fatigue really bothered me yesterday but today it feels a bit further away.'
- 'When the fatigue is around a lot, I feel more irritable.'

I have also seen many patients who use personalised language excessively, gradually merge their identity with the diagnosis. This can be a complex issue and not changed purely by use of language, but for starters:

> If you don't want the fatigue, don't call it yours.

The one who has knowledge uses words with restraint.
Book of Proverbs[NIV]

TIP 13: NOTE HOW THE FATIGUE AFFECTS ALL YOUR SYMPTOMS

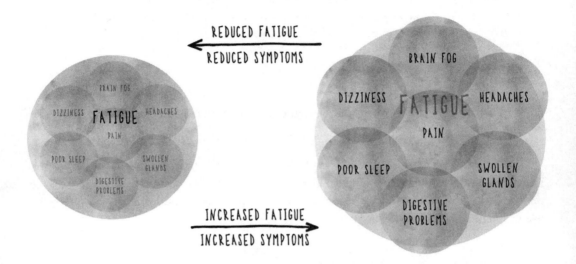

As the illustration shows, when the fatigue is reduced, all the accompanying symptoms are also reduced. Conversely, when the fatigue is particularly bad and dominating, all the other symptoms usually worsen as well. This is sometimes known as a 'flare-up' or a 'setback'.

When this occurs, some of the other symptoms can be shouting so loudly that they can direct all your attention and focus to them, to the exclusion of the fatigue. For example:

- Going to the hospital to get a headache checked out. The results are all clear, but the headache is still there. It takes days to recover from the exhaustion.

- Going to bed due to joint and muscle pain. The sleep cycle gets even more out of sync. It takes a few weeks to get it back to how it was.

- Unsettled stomach leads to not eating. Very low energy is experienced for days.

The above are examples only, but they demonstrate how focusing on one symptom, to the neglect of the overall fatigue management, only prolongs and exacerbates setbacks and flare-ups.

> Maintaining fatigue management strategies helps reduce all your symptoms.

- Take a moment to consider your own experience; in the coming weeks, be aware of your focus when other symptoms are demanding your attention.

> The pain of the little finger is felt by the whole body.
> Filipino proverb

TIP 14: REFLECT, REFLECT, REFLECT

When we see our reflection, it is natural to want to make some quick adjustments to our appearance, be it to flick our hair or straighten our clothing.

> Similarly, the more clearly you can see what is going on objectively, with your health and the fatigue, the easier it will be to make healthy adjustments.

There have been many times when I have sat with patients, and they have struggled to remember what they did that morning, never mind the previous week. As you practise the skill of reflection – pondering and thoughtfully considering all your activities and their effects on your health – you will be able to discern what direction your recovery is to take.

Life can be hard work when fatigue is present. During therapy sessions, I often felt as though we were 'panning for gold' in the midst of all the mud and dirt of life with fatigue.

> In other words, I wanted to facilitate finding some lesson or insight, or key, to potential ways forward from all the difficulties. Oftentimes that was in the very small details: the extra 5 minutes, the daytime nap, the long conversation, taking a moment each day to get some fresh air, the effects of an argument, and stopping to take rest breaks on the walk home. This may not sound like gold to you, but I assure you that the small insights and tweaks to activities in the coming days will make all the difference.

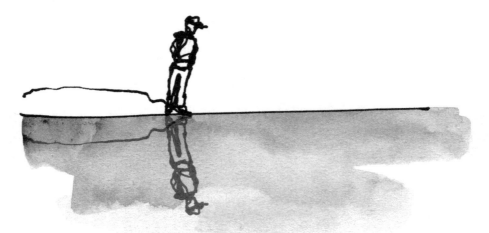

Therapy is not just about listening to how bad things are and repeating the same thing. It is trying to discern together what has worked, what has not, and what we can do differently to stay on the road to recovery.

I want you to make the most of every up and down and not waste the valuable lessons they contain. The only way to do this is to take time to look back, reflect and slightly adjust the way forward. Reflection takes time.

The best knowledge is to know yourself.
Welsh proverb

TIP 15: LEARN TO RECOGNISE THE 'BOOM AND BUST' PATTERN OF FATIGUE

The 'boom and bust' (or 'push and crash' as it is known in North America) pattern of fatigue is the up-and-down energy capacity that no doubt you have already experienced.

The boom: This is when you can function and perform some level of activity. Usually, your symptoms are less and you feel more able to attempt certain tasks.

The bust: This is when you are suddenly unable to function or perform activities, no matter how hard you try. Usually, all your symptoms are exacerbated, and you are forced to rest.

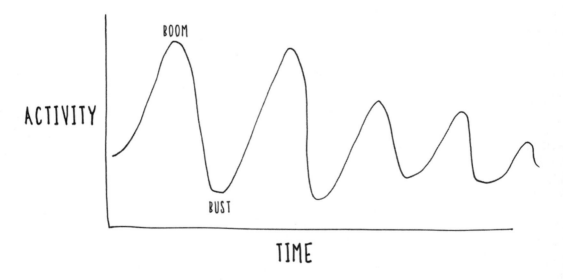

Let us consider the first boom peak on the graph. I am sure that if we had drawn this graph together before you became ill, your boom peak (activity capacity) would have been much greater – it would have been marked higher on the graph.

Whatever activity you engage in now, you can usually keep going until the fatigue and accompanying symptoms prevent you from continuing. This is then the bust (or crash). Usually, this is sudden and frustrating, and your whole body feels extremely fatigued. All your symptoms are exacerbated, and you are forced to rest. Some people describe this as 'having the plug pulled out', 'running out of petrol' or 'the light switch being turned off'.

Telling yourself to 'keep going' does not work. If it is possible to continue with that activity a bit longer, it only prolongs the bust/crash and makes it worse. Conversely, telling yourself to 'keep resting' all the time during the bust also prolongs that period and makes it worse. Rest is necessary but needs to be taken in healthy ways.

The boom and bust graph can be explained in terms of having a 'good day' followed by a 'bad day'. On a good day, symptoms are less and you may feel like catching up with some of the activities you are behind on. This overexertion on the 'good day' (boom) is then followed by a 'bad day' (bust) of enforced rest and the need to recover. This is also known as post-exertional malaise or 'PEM'.

However, with regard to the Time (x) axis on the graph, the unit of time may not be just a day. Depending upon the demands of the activity and your capacity, the time may be a few minutes or hours, a day, a few days, a week or a few weeks. The pattern of fatigue is the same and it will continue in this manner if left unchecked. You will also notice from the graph that, if left unchecked, your capacity will be reduced over time. This is the opposite of recovery.

In this process, it is important to learn to recognise this pattern in your own life. Think about a recent activity where you experienced boom and bust.

- How were you feeling at the start, middle and end of the activity?
- Be aware this week of the boom and bust pattern in your various daily activities.

Life is like a wheel, sometimes you are up and sometimes you are down.
Filipino proverb

TIP 16: TRY THE TRAFFIC LIGHT SYMBOL

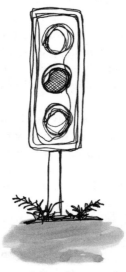

Once you recognise the boom and bust pattern of fatigue in your daily activities, it is important to spot the early warning signs for both the boom and the bust patterns before they occur.

Stop (Red)	=	Bust
Warning (Amber)	=	About to either boom or bust
Go (Green)	=	Boom

Usually, people can easily describe what they experience when they are on Go (Boom) or Stop (Bust), but it takes more skill and discernment to take heed of the Warning light.

Recognising those early warning signs in your body will help you make a choice, rather than be a victim of the fatigue. The Warning light prevents you from both booming/overdoing and also from busting/underdoing.

Here are a few examples of what these early warning signs may look like:

a. Go: Able to do computer work, no obvious symptoms.
    Warning: Sore eyes, dull headache starting.
    Stop: Complete brain fog, hard to think straight, need to rest.

b. Go: Enjoy a rare, short walk.
    Warning: Muscles aching in legs. Feel tired.
    Stop: Heavy painful limbs. Need complete rest.

c. Go: Enjoy seeing a few friends in a crowded, noisy environment.
    Warning: Struggle to focus on conversation. Sore throat, feel lightheaded.
    Stop: Difficulty saying words correctly. Swollen glands, feel hot and cold, need to lie down.

- Spend some time considering what some of your warning signs have been in different situations.

- Be attentive in the coming days to spot the warning signs.

A warning to the wise is a blessing.
Swahili proverb

TIP 17: USE AN ACTIVITY DIARY

A simple visual activity diary is a useful tool. It helps you understand the fatigue, as you reflect on the past week, and it guides you with the small changes needed to better manage and take control. It gives an overview of everything that demands your energy in your waking hours.

This is not a narrative diary, or a thoughts/feelings diary. Some people find it a chore to do because it can seem monotonous, but it is worth it.

I recommend doing it thoroughly for two weeks, then repeating it two months later and noting the difference. Choose your own rhythm and what works for you but do not do it continuously.

Everything that you do in a day takes physical, mental or emotional energy. Getting out of bed, washing, dressing, eating, reading messages on your phone, climbing the stairs, talking to a family member, planning a shopping list, responding to an email, watching TV, etc. Write, in hourly slots, the main activity you were doing in that hour. Try to fill it in on a daily basis.

Highlight the:

- low-energy activities
- medium-energy activities
- high-energy activities.

This is a subjective measure of what you consider to be low-, medium- or high-energy activities. This may vary from day to day depending upon how you are feeling and the situation. At the end of each day, score your fatigue levels for that day between 0 and 10, where 0 = no fatigue and 10 = maximum fatigue.

See Appendix 1 (page 268) for Activity Diary sheets.

After completing two weeks of activity diary sheets, ask yourself the following questions:

- What do I notice? What does that tell me?
- Where are the boom and bust patterns?
- Do the boom and bust patterns correlate with high, medium and low-energy activities and the fatigue scores?
- Do my days and activities look balanced? If so, what did I do well? If not, what could I have done differently?
- How can I change next week's activities to be more balanced and spaced out?
- Have I made any other observations?

Life can be understood backwards, but we live it forwards.
Swahili proverb

TIP 18: BEWARE OF THE SECONDARY ISSUES WITH FATIGUE

Chronic fatigue is identified as the primary or main issue. A secondary issue is something that has developed as a result of having chronic fatigue. This is understandable, and to be expected, with any form of chronic illness.

It is always useful to identify and name these secondary issues for what they are, on your journey to recovery. Sometimes they come for a season and then they go. Often they are resolved as the fatigue resolves.

At other times, especially when they are not acknowledged, they can grow and develop to become a more dominant issue than the actual fatigue. In other words, they become the primary issue and fatigue then becomes the secondary issue. You will see from the illustration that I have included some familiar symptoms of chronic fatigue such as sleep and pain. I have seen people recover well from chronic fatigue but still have disordered sleep, or persistent pain, as these have subsequently become the more dominant issue.

When this is the case, normal fatigue management strategies are limited in their effectiveness. These issues need to be acknowledged promptly and usually require attention.

In my experience, this is especially true with anxiety, relationship issues and deconditioning. Stop and consider:

- Are you aware of any secondary issues that are possibly getting in the way of your recovery?

- What do you think would help?

There is no cure for him who hides an illness.
Ethiopian proverb

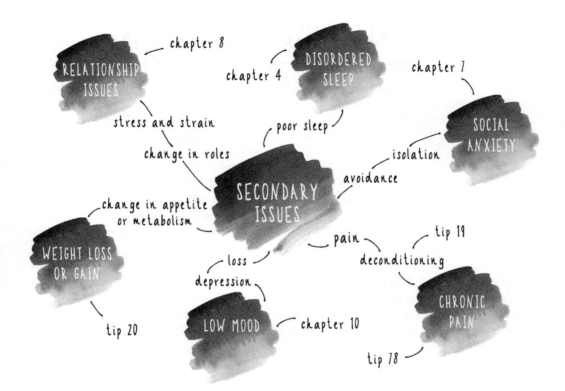

RELATIONSHIP ISSUES — chapter 8

DISORDERED SLEEP — chapter 4

SOCIAL ANXIETY — chapter 7

stress and strain

change in roles

poor sleep

isolation

avoidance

SECONDARY ISSUES

change in appetite or metabolism

WEIGHT LOSS OR GAIN

tip 20

loss

depression

LOW MOOD — chapter 10

pain

deconditioning — tip 19

CHRONIC PAIN

tip 18

TIP 19: RECOGNISE DECONDITIONING

Deconditioning is one of the body's responses to underuse or inactivity. Putting it in simple terms, the body becomes unfit. This is natural, given that the fatigue prevents normal levels of activity and functioning.

In the past, the awareness of deconditioning led to some controversial treatments for chronic fatigue, such as GET (Graded Exercise Therapy). This was a prescribed amount of exercise that was gradually increased. Patients often suffered days of recovery after exercise. The NICE guidelines[7] now recommend that exercise is not a treatment or a cure for CFS, and that patients should self-manage within their healthy limits.

I am certainly not an advocate for GET. However, I also am not an advocate for non-activity and total rest. We need strength, stamina, suppleness and skill for our bodies to be physically fit. However, fatigue affects all of these.

Suppleness is flexibility and I have witnessed many patients benefit greatly from doing simple stretches and healthy activity/exercise, within their limits, for only a few minutes at a time. Extension stretches can be useful, as fatigue often causes you to be in a flexed position, either sitting or curled up.

Some do their stretches on a bed, in a chair, standing up or lying on a floor. Some have a regular practice and discipline, such as Pilates. Others, during periods of prolonged sitting, have intentionally stood up, stretched and walked around at regular intervals. The key is to make it part of your day and see what works for you. The aim is to prevent deconditioning.

Better little than too little.
Cameroonian proverb

TIP 20: MAINTAIN A HEALTHY DIET

Fatigue has a way of affecting your diet and appetite. Maintaining a healthy diet is one way that you can help put fatigue in its place.

I am not a dietitian, so am unable to comment on specifics. However, I have witnessed much in relation to diet and fatigue over the years. Here are the main tips that I have seen work, along with points to consider:

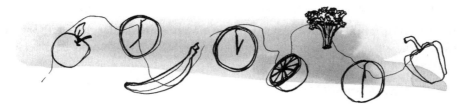

- Food is your fuel. If you don't put food into your body, you will not have the energy you need to function.

- Stick to regular mealtimes.

- If you experience a loss of appetite or feel overwhelmed when attempting to eat, serve smaller portions and have small healthy snacks in between meals. Work to gradually increase your portion size. Aim to keep mealtimes calm and relaxed.

- With some people, digestive and irritable bowel-type issues can be their most dominant symptoms. If that is your situation, continue to use the fatigue management strategies, as these will help to settle the symptoms.

- Avoid eating large meals late in the evening as this tends to disrupt sleep.

- If you eat too much 'junk' food, 'junk' is probably what you will experience.

- Limit your caffeine and sugar intake, which gives a quick rush of energy but then the energy suddenly comes crashing down. This is somewhat like the boom and bust pattern of fatigue, which you are seeking to balance out.

- Being overweight or obese causes fatigue. For some people, being less active, due to the fatigue, can increase weight. Also, take note if you are tending to comfort eat. Seek help with weight and balanced nutrition.

- Meal planning and shopping for a balanced diet take time and effort. Take the time needed to plan, or delegate if possible.

- I have seen numerous people attempt many and varied elimination diets, with many and varied results. What seems to work for one person doesn't always work for another.

- If you have a deficiency identified through blood testing, such as iron or vitamin D, your doctor will prescribe supplements. These will make a difference to your energy levels, so do take them.

- With regard to other supplements, do not purchase them without first doing your research. I have seen people invest financially in some miracle cure, only to be left wanting, whereas others have found something beneficial. Be aware of any 'quick fix' promises and don't neglect the fatigue management in the process.

- If a friend or family member asks if you want any help, accept the offer. Try asking them to cook or purchase a healthy meal for you, as that would be a wonderful time-saving gift.

- Drink plenty of water (Tip 47).

Which tip is the most relevant for you at present?

How are you going to start putting it into practice?

The body enjoys health when the stomach is well filled.
Hawaiian proverb

FOOD FOR THOUGHT

The following quote, reproduced with permission, is from the Health & Safety Executive website,[8] referring to workplace fatigue in the normal population.

> Fatigue results in slower reactions, reduced ability to process information, memory lapses, absent-mindedness, decreased awareness, lack of attention, underestimation of risk, reduced coordination, etc.
>
> Fatigue can lead to errors and accidents, ill-health and injury, and reduced productivity. It is often a root cause of major accidents e.g. Herald of Free Enterprise, Chernobyl, Texas City, Clapham Junction, Challenger and Exxon Valdez.
>
> Fatigue has also been implicated in 20% of accidents on major roads and is said to cost the UK £115 to £240 million per year in terms of work accidents alone.

Fatigue is something that is often not taken seriously enough.

PAUSE: STAR STRETCH

Try and stand in an open expansive stance, known as a 'star stretch'.
  You can also try this, sitting on a chair or lying in bed.
  If you are able, do this at frequent intervals throughout your day.

This stretch has many benefits:

- It counters the flexed body positions (sitting, lying curled up in bed) that the fatigue encourages.

- Some research[9] suggests that it can decrease your cortisol (stress) hormone by up to 25%.

- It may make you feel more confident and positive.

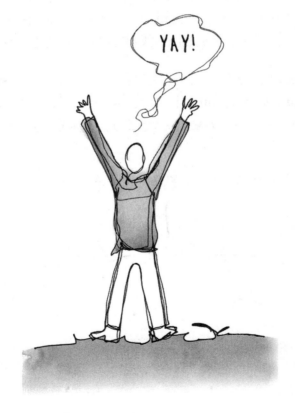

MIND, BODY AND SOUL: THE FATIGUE

Mind: What were your thoughts as you read this chapter on 'The fatigue'?

Other parts of the chapter you can let go of for now.

Body: What actions will you start putting into practice?

Soul: You may want to seek soul help with these changes.

As explained in the book's introduction, this section is from my perpective as a Christian, inviting God's help in the recovery process. You may have your own way of seeking soul help, so please do what you feel comfortable with.

Dear God, I ask you for help
with the fatigue and my recovery journey.
You say, – 'Come to me'.
'Come to me all you who are weary and burdened,
and I will give you rest ... rest for your souls.'[NIV]
Thank you, God.
Amen – may it be so.
Based upon Matthew 11[10]

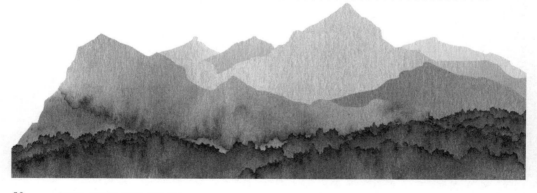

CHAPTER 3

SLEEP

It would seem to make logical sense that, if you suffer from fatigue, at least you would be able to have a good night's sleep, right? Well, as you have no doubt discovered by now, the fatigue does not play by the normal rules of life, and what your body is craving from a good night's sleep is sadly often denied.

As humans, we spend approximately a third of our lives sleeping. That is quite a lot of time. Sleep is essential for our mental and physical wellbeing. Sleep contributes to the proper functioning of our body's systems. Lack of sleep, therefore, has negative health consequences.

I have worked with many chronic fatigue sufferers who, although they sleep a lot, struggle to sleep *well*. From my experience, people either tend to over-think sleep issues, which can lead to increased anxiety about getting to sleep, or not to think enough about these issues, which can lead to disordered sleep habits.

Chronic fatigue sufferers who have sleep difficulties usually wake feeling unrefreshed. Some may not be waking until late morning or even into the afternoon. Often it is hard to get out of bed, as the body feels weighed down and heavy. The heavy feeling and sleepiness can continue throughout the day. Some people report feeling more alert for a few hours later on, often in the early evening. Almost a small window of hope, but this can be followed by difficulty switching off at night and not being able to get to sleep.

Changing your sleep pattern does not happen by chance. It does take a lot of patience, being intentional and very consistent. Concentrating on your sleep and developing healthy sleep hygiene habits together make the biggest difference to your overall health and ability to function and cope well. I have seen countless people transform their sleep habits and have witnessed the benefits. The change started when they chose to try something different.

Sleep difficulties can be complex and multi-faceted, but most can be solved. Ignoring sleep issues, and hoping they will go away, does not work. Trying to sleep for a few extra hours to fill the gap only tends to prolong the problems rather than solve them. When sleep is disordered, our bodies need to be retrained to know when it is time to sleep and when it is time to wake up.

What I have learnt over the years is that, even though some of these tips seem obvious, they almost need to be exaggerated, repeated and magnified in order to have an effect. Please keep that in mind as you start to put into practice the following tips, which will give you some useful starting points.

I have full confidence that you will benefit from healthier sleep habits.

TIP 21: SEPARATE DAY AND NIGHT CLEARLY

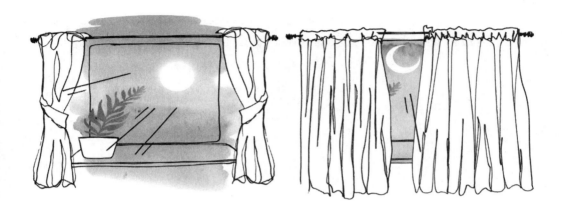

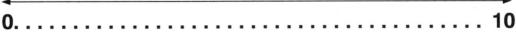

Daytime is for waking, night-time is for sleeping

This is probably not your present reality and that is okay for now, but please keep this fact clearly in your mind as a goal for your future sleep pattern. The boundaries between day and night can get very blurred with disordered sleep. The more disordered your sleep becomes, the more unrefreshing will be your experience. Reintroducing clear boundaries will prevent further deconditioning.

This is the direction we are heading towards to regain a healthier sleep routine. For now, just be aware of your current day and night sleep routine by drawing a line on the chart below where you think your sleep pattern currently is.

0 . . . . **10**

Sleeping a lot in the day   Sleeping only at night

In the weeks and months ahead, be aware of how your current line gradually changes position and consider what has contributed to that shift.

If you are sleeping excessively in the daytime and want to start changing that habit, see Tip 23.

> When you rise in the morning, give thanks for the light,
> for your life, for your strength.
> Native American proverb

TIP 22: KEEP A REFLECTIVE SLEEP DIARY

The reason for keeping a sleep diary is to understand your current sleep situation and give greater clarity to what may need to change. This sleep diary is more of a reflective diary rather than a scientific measurement of your sleep cycles (such as on a sleep app). A reflective diary can be more useful in empowering you to make some changes.

In your reflective sleep diary (see Appendix 2, page 276) consider the following questions:

- What was I doing an hour before bedtime?
- How was I feeling in the evening?
- What time did I get into bed?
- How long did it take me to fall asleep? Why? Any reasons?
- Did I wake in the night? How often? Why? Any reasons?
- What time did I wake up?
- What time did I get up?
- How did I feel?
- How would I rate my night's sleep out of 10? (10 being excellent.)

I would recommend only doing this for a week or two, no more than that. That is enough time to recognise any patterns of sleep and highlight any particular areas that need concentrating on.

Every few days, respond to the following statement:

If I could change the following, my sleep would improve:

1.

2.

3.

> Early sleep and early wake-up gives health
> and makes you grow.
> Portuguese proverb

TIP 23: SET AN ALARM

This tip is not always popular but it is of the utmost importance. When you are exhausted and perhaps have no particular reason to get up, it may seem sensible to rest for longer, but this is counterproductive. Staying longer in bed does not help poor quality sleep. Sufferers frequently report feeling worse for going back to sleep. Seeking balance and retraining your body to learn a sleep-wake cycle goes hand-in-hand with managing your activities, pacing and rest.

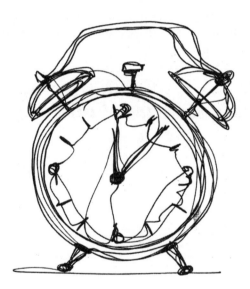

I recommend that you try the following method to create an ordered sleep-wake cycle:

- Decide what time you would like to wake and get up, for example 8.00 am.

- Use a simple alarm clock with a silent tick.

- Place the clock somewhere that requires you to move to switch it off.

- Check your reflective sleep diary and set the alarm for the average weekly time you currently wake and get up – for example, it maybe 11.30 am.

- Set your alarm at this time for a week, so that you get used to waking up with the alarm.
- Avoid going back to sleep – open the curtains, turn the light on, sit on the edge of the bed, put your pillows on the floor, etc.
- The following week, set your alarm for 30 minutes earlier.
- The following week, set your alarm for another 30 minutes earlier.
- Do this consistently for a few weeks, until you are waking and getting up at your preferred time.

If the 30-minute chunks are not successful, try 15-minute chunks of time.

> If your sleep is totally reversed – that is, most of your daylight hours are spent sleeping and your night-time hours are spent awake for weeks at a time – Tip 28 is more relevant to your situation.

No good will come of oversleeping.
Welsh proverb

TIP 24: USE YOUR BED FOR SLEEP ONLY

Some people use their beds for:

- Work
- Phone calls/social media
- Video games
- TV
- Eating food
- Putting their make-up on/styling their hair
- Socialising.

They then expect to be able to relax, switch off and sleep well.

This is especially true of teenagers, but many adults also fall into these unhelpful habits. When chronic fatigue comes along, clear boundaries need to be put back into place. Bedrooms need to be cleared of distractions, but also associations. If you have a habit of working on your bed, even when you sit there you will tend to think about work.

If you want to sort your sleep out: **use your bed for sleep only.**

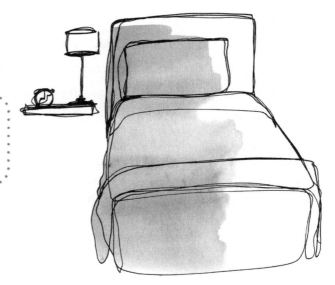

As you make your bed,
so you will sleep.
Russian proverb

TIP 25: ESTABLISH A BEDTIME ROUTINE

A bedtime routine is needed to retrain your body to know when it is time to switch off and go to sleep. It is important to exaggerate and prolong each step of this process. Keep repeating it until your body gets the message.

Points to consider are:

- Write out a realistic plan for your evening routine that is within your capacity and energy levels.

- Make it structured, relaxing and calming.

Depending upon your capacity, preferences and difficulties, your plan may look something like this:

9.00 pm:	Have a light snack and small drink, and sit for 5 minutes
9.20 pm:	Switch off the TV, all screens and devices
9.30 pm:	Go upstairs and sit for 5 minutes
9.40 pm:	Run a bath
9.50 pm:	Have a relaxing bath
10.10 pm:	Wrap yourself in a towel, sit for 5 minutes then get dressed for bed
10.20 pm:	Get into bed and dim the bedside light
10.30 pm:	Switch the light off.

Make a note of your reaction as you read the example above. It may help give you clues as to what might be useful or not for you to change.

Design your plan now. Write it out and try it. You may want to alter it slightly after a couple of days, but then try and do it consistently.

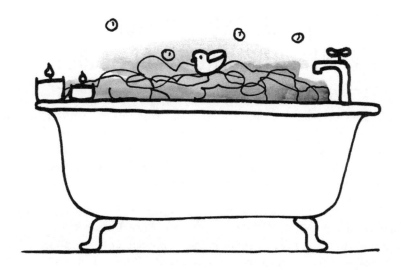

The loss of one night's sleep is followed by
10 days of inconvenience.
Chinese proverb

TIP 26: PROBLEM-SOLVE ENVIRONMENTAL SLEEP ISSUES

Sleep difficulties can be complex, multifaceted and frustrating. Approaching them with *simple* answers sometimes seems too simplistic. It can also appear that the gravity of the situation is not fully appreciated or taken seriously. I assure you that I am passionate about everyone getting a good night's sleep. We need our sleep. However, we can easily get into a bind about sleep issues and overlook the obvious.

Here are common-sense solutions to frequent sleep issues. There is nothing new in these lists, but they have all helped someone at some point to turn a corner. Look and see what draws your attention. Consider how you can start putting that into practice. Maybe you have some solutions of your own?

If you are unable to fall asleep after 20-30 minutes, get up and do something relaxing and unstimulating for a short while before attempting to fall asleep again.

a. *Light*

Our body naturally produces the essential hormone melatonin, also known as the 'sleep hormone'. It is responsible for telling our brains when it is time to wake up and when it is time to go to sleep. The light around us influences its production in our bodies.

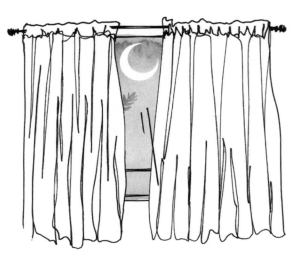

As darkness falls in the evening, melatonin production increases, causing the body to relax and feel sleepy. In the early hours of the morning, it decreases, causing the body to prepare and wake up and feel more alert. This cycle continues every day of our lives and it is the body's natural way to keep us healthy and facilitate refreshing sleep. Light, even for the shortest periods, interrupts this process and is detrimental to healthy sleep.

Possible solutions include:

- Consider all the artificial lights you use after sunset; take note and be aware.

- Use blackout blinds or curtain liners, especially in the summer months.

- Try soft eye masks, although they may take some getting used to.

- Use low-lighting lamps an hour before bedtime; consider having a sunrise/sunset stimulation-alarm lamp for your bedroom.

- Be ruthless and do not view screens for an hour before bedtime. (TVs, laptops, computers and phones use blue light.)

- Consider having a red nightlight on the landing and in the bathroom for night-time use.

b. *Noise*

Some people can sleep through anything and if that happens to be you, you are very fortunate.

Possible solutions include:

- Check your bedroom in the daytime and remove anything that makes the slightest noise; that could be chargers, phones, other devices. Do not share a room with pets. This may sound obvious, but I have worked with people with sleep difficulties and later discovered that the main culprit was a nocturnal animal.

- Earplugs: trial different sorts for comfort. These are useful if you are sharing a room with someone who snores. Please note that if you have primary caring responsibility, for a baby or small children, wearing earplugs is not advised.

- Consider which is the quietest room in your home, away from traffic noise, neighbours' noise and teenagers' noise, or from a sleeping partner. If space allows, consider changing your bedroom for a trial period.

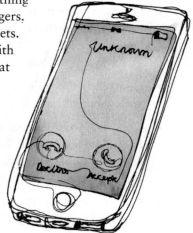

- If your finances allow it, purchase double or secondary glazing for your windows.

- Introduce a pleasant noise to your bedroom; some people have found the sound of a fan, or a trickling-water feature, soothing and relaxing throughout the night. You could also try sleep music or sleep stories.

c. *Comfort*

Have you ever heard people say, 'I can't wait to sleep in my own bed'? I have not heard that phrase recently during the pandemic as everyone has stayed at home, doing just that, but it implies that the traveller desires to return home and enjoy the comforts of their own bed, and the peace and rest that it gives.

Possible solutions include:

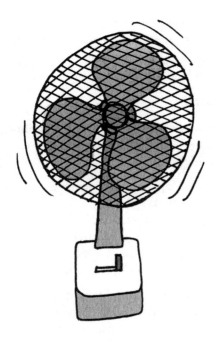

- Consider the position of your bed. Often there are not many options, but for some people having their bed moved to another position, if space allows, has helped significantly.

- Consider your bed frame. Does anything need repairing on the structure of the bed? Do any slats need straightening or replacing? Does the bed frame need tightening or oiling?

- Consider your mattress. Does it need turning? Does it sag in the middle? Does it need replacing? Would a mattress topper help?

- Consider your pillows. Try sleeping with some different pillows.

- Consider your sheets. How do they feel? How do they smell? Some people have found that non-fragrant detergent can counter their increased sensitivity.

- Consider your duvet and blankets, weight as well as temperature. Some people have benefited from a weighted blanket.

- Consider your nightclothes. Choose a material that feels cosy against your skin. Choose a size that allows free movement when turning in bed.

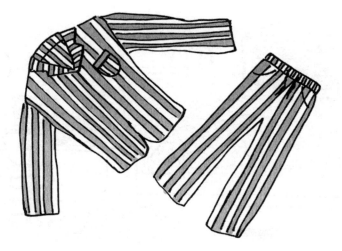

d. *Temperature*

Most people unknowingly keep their bedroom too warm, which causes restlessness and discomfort when sleeping. The ideal temperature is 18.3^{0}C (65^{0}F). During deep sleep, your body's ability to regulate temperature is reduced. This makes it more important to regulate the room's temperature, as well as the thickness of bedding, blankets and clothes. If the room is too cold, this can also interfere with sleep. Ventilate your room often.

e. *Atmosphere*

What is the atmosphere like in your bedroom right now? What do you sense when you walk into the room? Is it a place of calm and somewhere you can relax? Many people have difficulty sleeping because the atmosphere in their room is not conducive to it, maybe because it is:

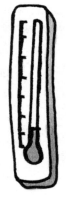

Cluttered: Unfinished projects, laundry that needs sorting, too many things in the room or items piled up that have no place to go.

Over-stimulating: Media, screens, music, as well as bold, eye-catching or emotive décor.

Work-based: Many of us have had to find a workplace at home, especially during the pandemic. If possible, avoid creating a workspace in your bedroom, or separate it by a screen if space allows. Tidy away all work-related items a few hours before bedtime.

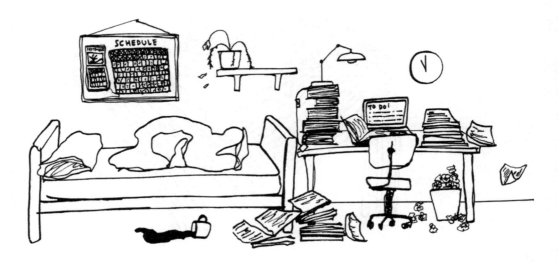

Dusty: No one can sleep well in an unclean space.

Changing a room can be a mammoth project. Try making small manageable changes in the short term. Spend time planning the larger changes and enlist help.

> If you think you are too small to make a difference,
> try sleeping in a closed room with a mosquito.
> African proverb

TIP 27: PROBLEM-SOLVE PERSONAL SLEEP ISSUES

As before, here are common-sense solutions to frequent sleep issues. There is nothing new in these lists, but they all have helped someone at some point to turn a corner. Look and see what draws your attention. Consider how you can start putting that into practice. Maybe you have some solutions of your own?

a. *Brain too active*

Over the years, many people have shared with me their frustrating stories of getting into bed physically exhausted but their mind almost being in overdrive. Obviously, getting frustrated about it only increases your adrenalin and alertness, keeping you wide-awake.

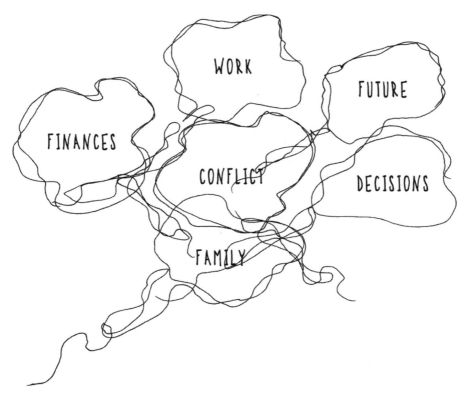

Sometimes the physical efforts of the day have demanded most of your attention and concentration; when your body is relaxing sometimes there can be more energy for thinking. Reflect on the last few occasions this occurred. Try to identify what you were thinking about. What themes were asking for your attention? Perhaps some themes may need additional support? If so, consider asking your doctor or healthcare provider for this. If the problem was overly active everyday thinking, then you probably need distraction techniques with something to focus your mind and attention on. This is where it is important to discover what works for you.

If you tend to have a visual creative imagination, try visualisation techniques. I know people who have put photographs of favourite places that evoke happy memories next to their bed. Some people have painted or drawn pictures that stimulate all their senses to enable them to relax – for example, imagining the warmth of the sun on their skin, feeling the sand between their toes, hearing the sound of the crashing waves, tasting ice-cream on their lips.

If you tend to have a more logical way of thinking, then while you are lying down, try to focus on a low-demand puzzle, such as a word search, Sudoku or 'spot the difference'. It needs to be relatively easy and somewhat boring. The aim is not to complete it but to focus your mind sufficiently until you are sleepy.

Other useful activities include:

- listening to calming music

- writing down your thoughts

- relaxation

- body scan scripts (see 'Pause: Mindfulness body scan practice for sleep' on page 78)

- reading a familiar book or magazine

- counting backwards from 1000.

If any of the mentioned activities makes you alert rather than sleepy, it is the wrong activity for you. Experiment and see what works.

b. *Digestive issues*

Various digestive issues can disrupt your sleep.

- Drinking too much fluid in the three hours before bedtime may cause you to need the toilet in the night; make sure you hydrate sufficiently earlier in the day.

- Eating a large meal late in the evening tends to cause indigestion; this often occurs when breakfast is skipped and meals are eaten in the afternoon and evening only. Where possible, eat regular meals at consistent times.

- Waking hungry at night: Again, this is usually because of disordered eating patterns.

In the very short term, you could have a snack by your bed to avoid waking fully. Concentrate on establishing your sleep and eating routine.

- Caffeine, a well-known stimulant. Avoid it and be aware that it is also in chocolate, so hot chocolate before bed is a bad idea, as are energy drinks in daylight hours.

- Alcohol may fool you into thinking that you are sleepy but it steals your deep quality sleep, only allowing you to sleep lightly; usually you wake up in the night, disrupting your sleep, when its effects have passed.

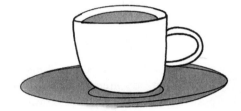

c. *Body not tired enough*

I have mostly heard this from people who are further down the road to recovery. They have put pacing into practice and now their body is recovering. In other words it can be a good sign.

Conversely, I have also heard it from people who are spending a lot of time in bed, which is not a good sign. They need to start introducing some structure and routine into their wake-sleep cycle.

To cut down on your daytime napping:

- Take extra preventative rests (Tip 51). Your body requires the right sort of rest.

- Keep curtains open and have some background noise on if napping.

- Sleep on the sofa for naps/rests, rather than your bed.

- Gradually cut back the duration and frequency of naps by setting an alarm or getting someone to wake you.

- Accept that you may feel worse as your body adjusts before you feel any better.

d. *Pain*

Having a warm bath, relaxation and body scan scripts can be useful. Just like chronic fatigue, pacing and activity management are priority treatments for chronic and persistent pain. Pain at night can be an indication of the need to balance the boom and bust cycle of activity. Sometimes, a specific medication for chronic pain and sleep can be useful, but only after healthy sleep routines and sleep hygiene have been attempted.

e. *Worry/stress*

If you regularly worry at bedtime, note down your concerns and leave them there to deal with in daylight hours; plan in a designated 'worry time' (see Tip 66) earlier in the day. Concentrate on a relaxing bedtime routine; use distraction techniques as outlined above.

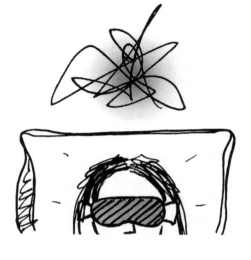

f. *Trauma/memories*

Waking up suddenly in a panicking state can be disturbing and frightening. If you have recently experienced a traumatic situation, your body will be on high alert, attempting to keep you safe and well from any perceived danger. It will take a while to soothe yourself to be calm enough and able to return back to sleep. At that moment, distract your attention onto your immediate surroundings; what you can hear, what you can see, what you can feel, what you can smell, what you can taste. Be kind to yourself and work on relaxing bedtime routines and extreme self-care (Tip 84, page 219).

Fear of dying from COVID and being admitted to hospital can evoke those feelings and emotions, as can past traumatic situations in your life. Time can often be a great healer, as can talking to people who can help with your fearful experiences. Talk soon to your healthcare provider, especially if this continues to/increasingly affects your sleep.

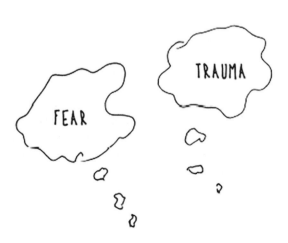

> An empty head gets the easiest sleep.
> Norwegian proverb

TIP 28: REVERSE SLEEP REVERSAL

Sleep reversal (or sleep inversion) is when most of your daylight hours are spent sleeping and your night-time hours are spent awake. It is not just for one or two days but usually for weeks at a time.

If your sleep is disordered *for only a few days*, Tip 23 is more relevant to your situation.

If your sleep is reversed for weeks at a time, give some consideration to how it became like this. Have you always tended to be alert and awake in the evening? What are the positives and negatives for you of having this kind of routine? Do you want to have a 'normal' or a different sleep routine? Do other people want you to have a 'normal' sleep routine, more than you do?

There is a reason why I ask these questions. In my almost 16 years of working in fatigue management, almost everyone has had some difficulties with sleep, yet only a small proportion of people had true sleep reversal. Frequently, but not always, other issues needed attention before they were in a position to work on changing the sleep reversal. Such issues included social anxieties, where being awake at night-time felt much safer

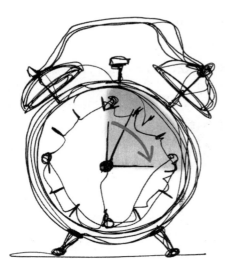

and more comfortable because no one else was around. This in turn led to avoidance of people in daylight hours. Once these issues are resolved you are in a better place to embrace a change in your sleep routine.

It is quite simple and reasonably quick to reverse sleep reversal. You need to set aside a week to dedicate the time to do it. The principle is that instead of trying to take your bedtime backwards (Tip 23), you stay up much longer and wake up later. It is crucial to have a routine and to stick to the bedtime and wake-up time. I have seen people do it in three-hour or four-hour blocks of time.

See the following example:

You have been going to sleep on average around 6.00 am and waking up around 4.00 pm for the last few weeks. This plan will take sleep forward in three-hour blocks.

	Bedtime	Wake-up time
Monday	6.00 am	4.00 pm
Tuesday	9.00 am	7.00 pm
Wednesday	12 noon	10.00 pm
Thursday	3.00 pm	1.00 am
Friday	6.00 pm	4.00 am
Saturday	9.00 pm	7.00 am
Sunday	9.00 pm	7.00 am

With this type of plan, you are more tired going to bed but you can still have the same amount of sleep.

All the other sleep tips in this chapter are important in this process. Be aware in your waking hours during this week, you may feel more tired than normal but stick to pacing, avoid all naps and use your alarm clock in the morning.

- Consider the questions posed at the start of this tip.

- Write a schedule and plan when you are going to start.

- Explain your schedule to someone who can support you during the week.

> One hour's sleep before midnight is better than three after it.
> French proverb

TIP 29: THINGS TO AVOID – THINGS TO TRY

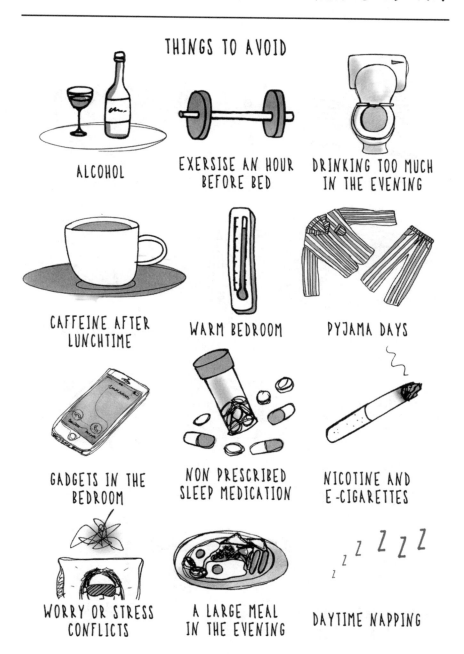

THINGS TO AVOID

ALCOHOL

EXERSISE AN HOUR
BEFORE BED

DRINKING TOO MUCH
IN THE EVENING

CAFFEINE AFTER
LUNCHTIME

WARM BEDROOM

PYJAMA DAYS

GADGETS IN THE
BEDROOM

NON PRESCRIBED
SLEEP MEDICATION

NICOTINE AND
E-CIGARETTES

WORRY OR STRESS
CONFLICTS

A LARGE MEAL
IN THE EVENING

DAYTIME NAPPING

THINGS TO TRY

READING IN BED

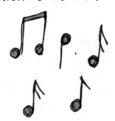

LISTENING TO CALM
MUSIC

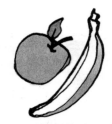

A SMALL NO SUGAR
SNACK

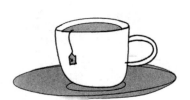

WARM MILK OR
HERBAL TEA

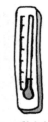

COOL BEDROOM

DAYTIME EXPOSURE
TO NATURAL LIGHT

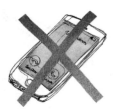

A GADGET FREE
BEDROOM

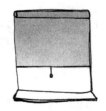

BLACK OUT BLINDS

ALARM CLOCK
WAKE UP LIGHT

SEE PAUSE

A RELAXING ACTIVITY
IF CAN'T SLEEP

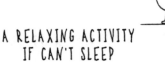

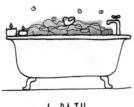

A BATH

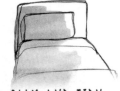

A CALM AND TIDY
BEDROOM

TIP 30: CHANGE YOUR NARRATIVE ABOUT SLEEP

When you are asked the question, 'How did you sleep?' what is your answer? I have asked this question countless times and the answer tends to be mainly negative. This still occurs when someone has made significant improvements with their sleep. Does this happen for you?

When family and friends enquire about your sleep, do you end up repeating and reinforcing the story of poor sleep? Maybe you don't, but just observe how you answer next time. The more the story gets repeated, the more fixed the narrative can become.

'I always sleep badly.'

'Terrible night's sleep, as usual.'

I am not an advocate for glossing over the truth, or for avoiding your current reality. Far from it, but I have seen the detrimental effects of continually focusing on the difficulties and negatives. No change takes place when this is the case. The small exceptions to the dominant-problem narrative get overlooked. Those small exceptions are part of the change that you are longing for. Don't ignore them. Don't disregard them. Try amplifying them. Try focusing on them. Try exaggerating them. Try talking about them.

If you are asked the question, 'How did you sleep?' an alternative answer could be to pause and think of at least one positive about the previous night's sleep.

'I didn't need to get up last night.'

'Even though I only slept for a short time, I was not in pain.'

'It didn't take me as long to get off to sleep.'

'I struggled to switch off, but I was able to distract myself.'

'I didn't wake as often as the night before.'

'Even though I didn't feel like it, I woke with the alarm.'

Thinking and talking about these small positives will certainly position you for a better start to the day.

Suggest a replacement question to be asked such as, 'What went well last night?' rather than, 'How did you sleep?' Replacement questions, such as this, position you to change your narrative about sleep.

He who cannot sleep can still dream.
African proverb

FOOD FOR THOUGHT

Matthew Walker, in his compelling book *Why We Sleep*[11] concludes with these inspired remarks:

I believe it is time for us to reclaim our right to a full night of sleep, without embarrassment or the damaging stigma of laziness. In doing so, we can be reunited with the most powerful elixir of wellness and vitality, dispensed through every conceivable biological pathway. Then we may remember what it feels like to be truly awake during the day, infused with the deepest plentitude of being.*

z z Z Z Z

---

*With kind thanks to Matthew Walker and his publishers for these words

PAUSE: MINDFULNESS BODY SCAN PRACTICE FOR SLEEP

Mindfulness meditation is something we can all do to support our health and wellbeing. It simply involves paying attention in the present moment and doing so with an attitude of kindness towards ourselves. The intention of any mindfulness practice is to 'fall awake' to what is happening inside us and outside of us. Sometimes, mindfulness can help promote relaxation, reduce stress and improve the quality of sleep, particularly when practised before going to bed. The following guided meditation may help this happen for you.

Start by choosing a comfortable position that will enable you to rest and relax, perhaps lying down on your bed with a cover over you for warmth.

Your intention for this practice is simply to pay attention to your body, scanning for any noticeable sensations, such as vibration, tingling, heaviness, lightness, pressure, space, movement, heat, coolness and contact with your bed, your clothing and the air that surrounds you. Within the body scan, your practice is to simply acknowledge these sensations without trying to change them, by being curious about them and open to experiencing them in the present moment.

During the body scan you may notice that you become distracted by competing sensations, thoughts or arising emotions that take your attention away from the practice. This is normal. Your practice is to acknowledge where your mind has wandered to, and then to let go by gently, but firmly, redirecting your focus back to your breathing and to your body.

1. **To begin the meditation, focus your attention on your breathing.** Notice where you feel your breath in your body. Perhaps you can feel the coolness of the air as it grazes the top of your lip on the in-breath, and the warmth of the outward breath? Perhaps you can feel the rise and fall of your chest, or the expansion and release of your abdomen as you breathe in and out? Remember, your breath is always there for you as a safe place to return to should you feel unsettled in any way.

2. **Now move your attention to the top of your head.** Notice the contact of your head with the pillow beneath it, and any sensations across your scalp. Can you feel your hair follicles? What are you experiencing? Be curious.

3. **Gently guide your focus down onto your face.** Allow your attention to focus on sensations across your forehead, around your eyes, at your nostrils, in your ears, at your lips, in your mouth and along the length of your jaw. What do you notice? Any tension, tightness or clenching? Just see whether you can let this go on an outward breath? Is there any sense of release?

4. **Now move your awareness down into your neck to come to settle in your shoulders.** What do you notice here? Any sense of tension, heaviness or weight? Can you feel your shoulder joints and any areas of contraction or tiny areas of space? Just be curious about what is here.

5. **Allow your focus to travel down into both arms and hands.** Tune in to any arising sensations in the muscles of your upper arms, elbows, wrists, fingers and thumbs. Can you feel tingling? Pulsing? Vibration? See whether you can focus on feeling your arms and hands from the inside, experiencing the long muscles, and the complex joints. If your arms and hands could speak, what would they say to you?

6. **Guide your attention back up to come to rest in your chest and abdomen.** Notice how your chest moves with the breath in your body. See whether you can tune in to your heart, encased behind your rib cage, and the space that surrounds it. What do you notice? Any clenching? Or perhaps a sense of relief from being exactly who you are in this moment? What do you notice in your abdomen? Is there a sense of fullness or hunger? Simply pay attention.

7. **Allow your focus to travel back to the tops of the shoulders and to roll down into your back.** What sensations are arising at the top of your shoulder blades? See if you can follow the path of your spine downwards, taking in the curve of your backbone and the contact your body has with the surface on which you are lying. Explore the upper back, the middle of your back and the lower back where you may store tension. Experiment with releasing into the bed a little more with each out-breath.

8. **Guide your attention into the pelvic girdle.** The invitation is to become aware of all the delicate organs encased in this boney structure and to explore any sensations that may be arising here. Is there heaviness? Contraction? Lightness? Space?

9. **Now softly move your focus to come to settle in both hips.** Rest in an awareness of both hip joints and all they do for you each day; how they enable you to bend, to sit, to stand and walk. What do you notice here?

10. **Gently move your attention down into both legs.** Explore the long thigh bones and the long loose muscles. What sensations do you feel? Can you let go a little further and allow the legs to roll out to the side?

11. **Allow your awareness to then settle on both of your knees.** Be curious about any arising sensations across the tops of your kneecaps and in the soft underside of the knees. Can you experience the connection your knees have with your thighs and calves beneath them?

12. **Lightly focus your attention on your lower legs now.** Explore your calf muscles and shin bones. Can you feel the stretch of your skin across the bones? Can you feel the softness of the contact beneath you? Is there any sense of warmth or coolness?

13. **Guide your focus down into your ankles, feet and toes.** Investigate any sensations here. This is perhaps an area of the body you only notice when it is causing some discomfort. What do you feel? Any tingling sensations across the soles of the feet? Any contact with the material that covers you?

14. **Now allow your awareness to slowly widen out to include a sense of the whole of your body lying here in stillness.** Notice your breath moving within you. Observe how the body breathes itself without any conscious involvement from you. Rest here for as long as you like, and as well as possible; invite in a sense of gratitude and kindness towards your body, for all that it does for you day-to-day; this body is the only one you have.

15. **You have now come to the end of the body scan.** If you wish, you can start again and scan through your body as many times as you like. You may even want to experiment with beginning at your feet and going up to the top of your head this time. [†]

HAPPY PRACTISING!

---

† With kind thanks to Linzi Bound, Mindfulness teacher, for these words.

MIND, BODY AND SOUL: SLEEP

Mind: What were your thoughts as you read this chapter on Sleep?

Other parts of the chapter you can let go of for now.

Body: What actions will you start putting into practice?

Soul: You may want to seek soul help with these changes. As explained in the book's Introduction, this section is from my perspective as a Christian, inviting God's help in the recovery process. You may have your own way of seeking soul help, so please do what you feel comfortable with.

Dear God, I ask you for help with my sleep
and my recovery journey.
'I lift up my eyes to the mountains.
Where does my help come from?
My help comes from the Lord, the maker of heaven and earth.
He who watches over you will not slumber.
The Lord will watch over your coming and
going both now and for evermore.'[NIV]
Thank you God.
Amen may it be so.
Based upon Psalm 121[1,2]

CHAPTER 4

MINDSET – MOTIVATION

No doubt, chronic fatigue has brought about changes that you have not welcomed or wanted, and yet more change is required for recovery. Over the years, I have witnessed that change occurs gradually. It is rarely easy and generally requires a gradual progression of small steps towards recovery. Relapses are part of the process and that is okay. Each step takes you closer to your preferred future. Motivation involves wanting to change. When you are motivated, you are energised to bring about that change by being persistent with your actions and new habits.

> Did you know that, according to experts, it takes more than two months to form new habits?[13] Recovering from this horrendous illness is all about forming new habits, little by little, taking baby steps. Staying motivated is vital in order to keep going healthily with that process.

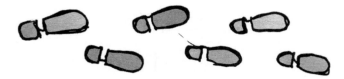

Intrinsic, or internal, motivation is when you are compelled to do certain actions because you want to or they are important to you personally – why you choose to do certain activities over others or what your passions, desires and interests direct you towards. Extrinsic, or external, motivation is when you are compelled to do certain actions because of external factors or circumstances. Both types are useful in enabling you to take steps forward.

Over time, psychiatrists and psychologists have studied motivation, recognising the important part it has in recovery. Three useful visual models that I have sometimes used in my work are:

- The Process of Transition Curve[14] (John Fisher)
- The Stages of Change Model[15] (or the Transtheoretical Model)
- The Five Stages of Grief[16] (the Kübler-Ross Model)

I have worked with all levels of motivation, ranging from complete opposition to the idea of pacing and fatigue management, to being highly motivated to get started. So wherever you find your motivation levels today, they can and often do change. Motivation is required each step of the way, so it is important to be informed and take steps to maintain this for your recovery journey. Motivation lightens and facilitates the road ahead. In this chapter, we will consider tips to stay motivated.

TIP 31: KNOW YOUR 'WHY' AND SEEK INSPIRATION

What is your motivation for engaging in fatigue management strategies?

It may be:

- to have more energy and capacity.
- to regain some of what has been lost.
- to be able to think clearly again.
- to be able to get back to work, school or college.
- to be able to enjoy being around people.

Or it may be for some other reason.

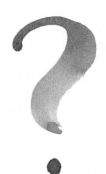

What is your 'why'?

Jot down a few reasons now as this will help
encourage you when you need it.

I have seen the power of people's stories in motivating and encouraging others who are also struggling with chronic fatigue. When you hear a story that is so familiar to your own, it can feed your soul in ways nothing else can. Firstly, it makes you realise that you are not going mad, as it validates your own experience and makes you feel less isolated. Secondly, you can glean what has worked for the other person and what has not. They have done a lot of the hard work on your behalf. Thirdly, it can give you hope and motivate you to prioritise recovery.

One regret from my working life was that I did not capture more of those stories in a written or media format. Many people who recovered would have wanted their journey to inspire others, but, as with most NHS professionals, the needs of a busy caseload diverted my attention from capturing those powerful testimonies. Most of the stories in the general media domain are of current sufferers rather than people who have recovered or are in the process of recovering from CFS/ME or long COVID. This is understandable given the severity and enormity of chronic fatigue and the relatively recent development of long COVID.

Role models can often inspire us in life when there is perhaps a lack of testimony-type stories. They have gone before or are people we admire because of their achievements or character traits. They could be people we know personally, fictional characters or famous people but, whoever they are, something about them enriches our life and provides us with hope, motivation and encouragement.

- Who are some of your role models?

- What might they say to you today?

- What encouragement do you gain from them?

Examples often do much more than words and teachers.
German proverb

TIP 32: GOALS – THINK SMALL, DREAM BIG

Most literature on motivation clearly outlines the importance of having a clear vision with aims and goals. When the going gets tough, these enable you to persevere and not quit. In the context of this rehabilitation journey, they enable you to keep applying fatigue management strategies to have an increased capacity and a healthier life.

Setting goals or considering big dreams for the future involves being hopeful that things may and can change. You may or may not be in a place of too much hope right now and that is okay. Your goals and dreams will probably reflect the hope you are currently experiencing.

Some people enjoy the whole process of goal setting and other people hate it. For those who enjoy it, there are many tools available to assist you. Find a method that suits your preferences.

One such simple tool is SMART goals:

SPECIFIC – What, Why and How?

MEASURABLE – Short-term goal, set to know when it is achieved.

ATTAINABLE – The goal is practical and possible.

REALISTIC – The goal is within reach, given your situation.

TIME-LIMITED – Enough realistic time to reach the goal.

For those of you who are not a fan of goal setting (I have met many), answering open-ended questions can be a useful start:

- How do you picture your life in two years' time?
- What areas do you want to grow in or develop?
- What could be the first step?
- When you have more energy, what activities will be at the top of your list?

- If you could do anything now, what would it be?

For some people, the Miracle Question from Brief Solution-Focused Therapy[17] (see Food for thought in this chapter, page 100) is a useful tool. For others, simply keeping a picture on the wall of their ambitions or dreams is sufficient in helping them stay focused and motivated.

The greatest thing, in my opinion, that dashes motivation more than anything else is unrealistic goals and expectations. I have heard hundreds of people, over the years, discuss their plans for practical steps forward. Frequently my response has been, 'Cut it in half!'

I am not saying that is the right response to everything, but the majority of people tend to expect too much of themselves within a short period, as do professionals, relatives, work colleagues and managers, teachers and education staff, unless they have had prior experience of this condition.

Keep the dream alive with small, consistent, manageable steps which are the key to progress.

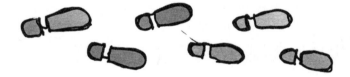

A journey of a thousand miles begins with a single step.
Chinese proverb

TIP 33: CONSIDER ACCEPTANCE

Acceptance of a diagnosis or medical condition, such as long COVID or chronic fatigue syndrome, and its implications and uncertainties, can vary enormously from person to person. Obviously, it can vary from day to day too.

The visual scale below may help you to position yourself in moving towards Active acceptance, as you grapple with your present reality and all the unanswered questions you may have.

Notice and become increasingly aware of a range of
thoughts and emotions, including discomfort

Non-acceptance	Active acceptance	Passive acceptance
Conflict	'It's okay for now'	Passivity
Resistance	Motivated	No progress
Searching for cause/cure	Seeking consistency	*It is what it is*
Minimal progress	Engaging with rehabilitation	*Just have to live with it*

- What is your present reality?

- Where would you put yourself on the scale?

- What might help you to move towards active acceptance?

> When the wind of change blows, some build walls
> while others build windmills.
> Chinese proverb

TIP 34: GIVE PRIORITY TO RECOVERY

Adjusting and adapting to fatigue management strategies takes time and can be costly. Time spent on your health needs to become a top priority for this season. It is time well spent.

> I have seen numerous people understand the principles of fatigue management but choose to prioritise other things. They are always important things, such as education, work, career and commitments. However, the longer-term effects of choosing other things over your health, *in this season*, usually make the process of recovery longer than it could have been.

Time taken for recovery is different for everyone, but I have noticed that people who make the process a priority appear to be more motivated and able to recover more quickly from setbacks. With time, they have recovered their health and wellbeing, and gone on to lead fuller lives and pick up some of their previously-held priorities.

A frequent objection to this tip is that some people do not feel that they have a choice. Is that how you feel? If so, consider what the objection to that choice is really saying. For example, 'I can't do that because...' often reveals something that is either a greater priority to you, or to someone else.

What areas do you have choices in? What will help or hinder you in making those choices? Consider how you can delegate, or shelve, something to a later date. There is always a choice, no matter how small or how costly. It could be the choice that makes all the difference.

- What priority is your recovery in this season?

- What choices are before you?

- What practical choice can you make today to prioritise your recovery in this season?

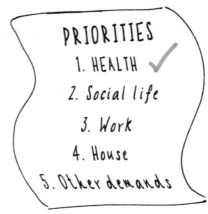

PRIORITIES
1. HEALTH ✓
2. Social life
3. Work
4. House
5. Other demands

Wisdom is like honey — if you find it
there is a future hope for you.
Book of Proverbs[NTV]

TIP 35: CELEBRATE EVERY SMALL ACHIEVEMENT

The steps to recovery from the fatigue can be so small and slow that you can totally miss them. That may sound ridiculous, but it is true.

Life, at times, can feel somewhat overwhelming with the fatigue. It is natural to focus on what you are struggling with and unable to do, but if that is your focus then that is all you will tend to see. This can be demoralising and at times make you wonder, 'What is the point?' You can easily get discouraged if you look too far ahead or too far behind at all the things you are not able to achieve at present.

Picture yourself saving up for an annual holiday. How would you feel if, in one month, you had managed to save 10% of the money? Personally, I would feel quite pleased, and I think you might do too. Maybe next month you could save 5%, or even 25%, but it would all be going towards your goal of having the money needed to purchase your holiday. Now picture your health. Do you have a sense of gratitude for the 5% recovery, or will you focus on the 95% deficit?

Frequently, with our health needs, we focus on the deficit and miss the tiny steps of progress. Progress can take a long time. When we celebrate even small achievements, it can have powerful effects on our brain. Not only does it cause endorphins, our 'feel-good' hormones, to be released, but it also teaches us to want to repeat that experience, thus reinforcing motivation. There is nothing more motivating than seeing that your efforts are reaping rewards and moving you in tiny steps towards your desired future.

In the early stages of recovery, the small steps of progress may, for example, be:

- having a shorter nap.
- taking more regular breaks.
- enjoying a phone conversation.
- experiencing more balance.

You will miss seeing these small wins if you are not looking for them. Avoid writing diaries that focus on your symptoms or how bad the situation is. You can stay motivated and learn so much by reflecting on every small achievement.

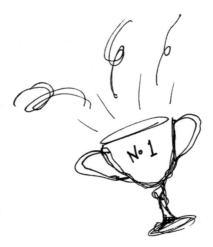

> At the end of each day, and week, ask yourself: *'What went well?'*

Even during difficult times, find something that went well. Celebrate it in some way to amplify it and remember it. By doing this often, you are training yourself to look for the exceptions within the problem narrative. This in turn will help you to stay motivated and focus on your recovery.

Even a little is more than nothing.
Hungarian proverb

TIP 36: DON'T LET YOUR EMOTIONS KNOCK YOU OFF COURSE

On this recovery journey you no doubt have had, and will continue to experience, many varied emotions. Your emotions and your response to them can change from moment to moment and day to day. Also your capacity to hold and manage these varied emotions is reduced at present. It is normal at times to feel overwhelmed, and equally normal at times to feel quite numb too.

Emotions are often what give life variety and colour. They can take us on highs and lows. Sometimes our emotional language – our ability to put into words our feelings – is not sufficient to express the range of emotions or the meanings they may hold for us. Emotions are often considered to be experienced in isolation within an individual's body. This is true but they are far richer than that. They are also relational in nature and a form of communication with, and an invitation to, others to respond.

The following illustration captures some of the emotions you might experience with chronic fatigue as you move towards your preferred, healthier future. Some can fuel your motivation, while others can completely drain it.

- Which emotions can you currently identify with?

- How do those emotions influence your engagement in fatigue management?

- How does stepping back, and seeing those emotions as part of the overall change and transition process, enable you to stay motivated?

If you are building something and a nail breaks, should you stop building altogether, or should you change the nail?
African proverb

AWKWARD

CHEERFUL

AWFUL

CAUTIOUS

CALM

JOYFUL

DISTRESSED

CRUSHED

FLAT

DESPONDENT

OPTIMISTIC

ANXIOUS

TENSE

DISCOURAGED

DEFENSIVE

BUOYANT

SHAME

FRIGHTENED

FEARFUL

DISILLUSIONED

CONTENTED

SORROWFUL

DISAPPOINTED

DISPIRITED

STRENGTHENED

DENIAL

GROUCHY

MAD

GUILTY

ACCEPTING

INDECISIVE

LIVID

ANNOYED

AGITATED

NUMB

DEPRESSED

SHY

ENCOURAGED

CONFIDENT

APPREHENSIVE

ECSTATIC

HAPPY

ENRAGED

WEEPY

ANGRY

EMBARRASSED

UNSURE

DETERMINED

FED UP

TIP 37: CONSIDER A SUPPORT TEAM

Anyone who appears to be successful in life usually has a great support team behind them. They are not always seen or known, but they are there, and they are real.

Just stop and think about a successful person in public life – it may be a sportsperson, politician or musician. Think about all the people behind the scenes who support that person in their current role. There could be coaches, trainers, managers, physiotherapists, dietitians, secretaries, assistants, scriptwriters, aides, advisors, chauffeurs, roadies and publicists, not to mention family, friends, neighbours and fans.

> We all need support and encouragement in life. When you suffer from chronic fatigue, and you start to learn how to manage it, it is important to have some support. Only *you* are responsible for your self-management recovery from chronic fatigue; nobody can do it to you. It is a hard, and often lonely, journey at times, especially when you are trying to change some of your habits. Your support team is therefore essential to encourage and cheer you on. It could include friends, family members, medical personnel, fellow sufferers, neighbours and people in your community.

Support could come from following the Pacing Group Guidelines (Appendix 3, page 278).

Often, people from your support team may not be available. A useful way to consider their encouragement and support is to picture them standing with you and ask yourself: 'What would ... say to me right now?'

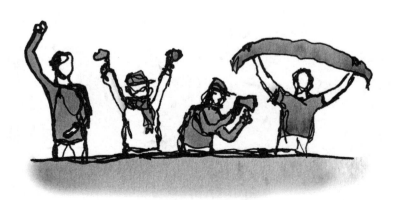

- Who would you consider to be on your support team?

- Picture them standing beside you.

- What do you appreciate about their support and contribution?

> When you see a turtle on top of a fence post,
> you know he has had some help.
> African proverb

TIP 38: BE KIND TO YOURSELF

What does it mean to *'be kind to yourself'*? It is a well-used phrase but it has multiple meanings and different connotations for different people. Practising it is harder than saying it.

- What does it mean for you?
- What does 'be kind to yourself' look like in practice for you?

Struggling with a chronic illness requires prioritising your health needs in order to recover. For some of you, shifting your attention onto yourself can feel somewhat uncomfortable and selfish and yet for others, this may come more naturally. We are not talking about being overindulgent or selfish. This is about treating yourself with kindness as you journey for the long haul, learning through trial and error.

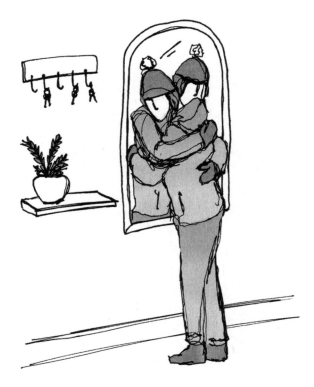

Kindness implies being:

forgiving	thoughtful	helpful
considerate	generous	sympathetic
supportive	gentle	compassionate
friendly	warm hearted	not harsh.
caring	charitable	

- Which words stand out for you?
- What helps you to be kind to yourself? What hinders you?
- What is one thing you can do today to be kind to yourself?

> Kindness is a language which the blind can see and the deaf can hear.
> African proverb

FOOD FOR THOUGHT

The 'Miracle Question' is part of Brief Solution-Focused Therapy.[17] For some, it may sound strange but I have seen this question motivate numerous people over the years. It can offer possibilities of hope and vision for a better future in beautiful ways. It is not for everyone and for some, as they become aware of loss, it can at times be painful.

Some people choose to capture their answers in a drawing or written form. The more details you can furnish the answer with, the richer your experience will be.

I want you to be creative in your thinking, as I ask you the Miracle Question.

Imagine that you have finished reading this page, put the book down and carried on with your day. When you go to sleep tonight, your home is quiet and something amazing happens as you sleep peacefully – a miracle happens.

Your fatigue and all related symptoms have completely gone. You are asleep and not yet aware that this miracle has occurred.

You wake in the morning. To your surprise, you feel different. You cannot explain it. You start to get out of bed...

Imagine that is your situation. Now describe in as much detail as you can:

- What is the first thing you notice as you are waking up?
- How do you feel?
- What do you sense?
- What can you do that you couldn't do yesterday?
- What are you thinking?
- How are things different?
- What differences do others notice about you?
- How does it affect your day's activities?
- How is your mood?
- How are your energy levels?

Use this picture of yourself in the coming days as inspiration to fuel motivation and set manageable goals.

PAUSE: HOBBIES

Is there an area of interest you would like to pursue? Maybe it is something completely new to you? Or something you have always wanted to do, but never had the time.

Many people affected by chronic fatigue spend their energy on just trying to live. Frequently many previous leisure or recreational activities are no longer possible. They used to give pleasure, enjoyment and social contact. This can, at times, leave a huge void.

Sometimes hobbies can give you a small sense of control and influence when a lot of your life does not feel in your control. I have noticed the motivation and energy-giving shift that can occur when people start to develop new hobbies or interests.

Often these new interests are started by reading magazines, watching more TV programs or Internet clips of 'How to…'. These can be developed in very small steps and within your time frame. They are usually more sedentary activities and can easily be picked up and put down.

Nelson Mandela[18] spent 27 years as a prisoner. He had to adjust to life with all the restrictions and limitations that prison life brought whilst, at the same time, maintaining hope and longing for his freedom. Whilst in prison, he learnt to garden and experienced great pleasure when he planted seeds in a small patch of earth and watched them grow. There was an element of freedom and a sense of control in being able to tend this allotment, observe seedlings grow and later pick the crops.

> Are there any interests or hobbies that you might like to pursue?
>
> What could be a small starting step?

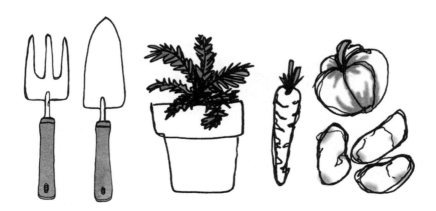

MIND, BODY AND SOUL: MINDSET — MOTIVATION

Mind: What were your thoughts as you read this chapter on Motivation?

Other parts of the chapter you can let go of for now.

Body: What actions will you start putting into practice?

Soul: You may want to seek soul help with these changes. As explained in the book's Introduction, this section is from my perspective as a Christian, inviting God's help in the recovery process. You may have your own way of seeking soul help, so please do what you feel comfortable with.

Dear God, I ask you for help with my motivation
and my recovery journey.
You say – 'I will lead the blind by ways they have
not known, along unfamiliar paths I will guide them;
I will turn darkness into light before them and make
the rough places smooth. These are the things I will do.'[NIV]
Thank you, God.
Amen – may it be so.
Based upon Isaiah 42[19]

CHAPTER 5

ENERGY

No doubt we have all had the experience of trying to use our phone, just when the battery goes flat. No amount of effort, or self-will or wishful thinking, will reconnect the phone and cause it to work. It needs to be recharged to function properly again.

The energy we need for our bodies to function fully can be considered in a similar light. With chronic fatigue, the amount of energy you have is significantly reduced. Your capacity, for now, is nothing like it used to be. This often leads to many situations where your energy just runs out and you are left wanting.

> This phenomenon is difficult to put into words - to express the full extent of how you feel whenthis sudden lack of energy and capacity occurs. I have heard many descriptive metaphors from other people's experiences of this:

'Like a light switch being turned off'

'Like a plug being pulled out'

'Like a car battery being flat — just can't get started again'

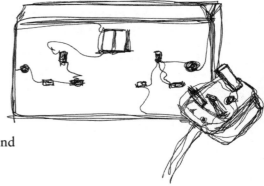

'Like my body is a ton weight, all of a sudden, and I can't move'

'Nice house – no one at home'

'Like a torch battery – weakly flickering on and off'

How would you describe your experience?
Do you have any metaphors that you find useful?

In this chapter, we will consider your energy capacity and the different types of energy:

- Physical energy
- Cognitive energy
- Social/emotional energy.

Often people only think in terms of physical energy but it is vital we understand cognitive and social/emotional energy too if we are to get good at regulating our energy levels. Most of the activities we perform in life use a combination of all these energy groups, but, for now, it is useful to consider each group separately. We will also consider the different ways you spend your energy.

TIP 39: RECOGNISE LIMITED CAPACITY

Picture your energy as coins stored in a 'piggy bank'. For every action, you pay with some of the energy coins. Some activities are more costly than others. You only have so many coins allocated for a particular day – no more, no less. When they are spent, you do not have a reserve of additional savings. There is no more.

Prior to becoming ill with this horrendous fatigue, your piggy bank was bigger and more flexible. In fact, for some of you, it was enormous and felt limitless. You could push the accelerator in life, overextend yourself on occasions and have the ability to bounce back. Lack of energy hardly ever curbed your activities. For others, maybe you had some prior limitations and restrictions, so your piggy bank would not have been enormous but it was probably much larger than it is now.

Your capacity or energy supply is significantly reduced at present. Your current piggy bank is smaller than you would like it to be; it is not the size it used to be. Some of your energy coins are only for physical activities, some are only for cognitive activities and others are just for social and emotional activities. For this season, you need to be wise and aware of how you spend each coin.

People often forget that everyday activities, such as getting washed, dressed, and making a phone call, all cost energy. You need to be able to spread out the coins throughout your day.

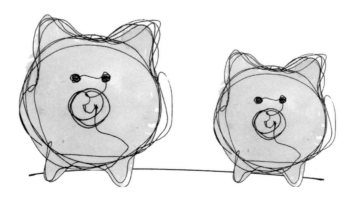

No doubt you desire to have a greater capacity, which will come with continued fatigue management. At this point, recognise and be aware of your current capacity.

Times change and we change with them.
Latin proverb

TIP 40: CONSIDER PHYSICAL ENERGY

Physical energy is used for any activity with your body.

That may sound obvious and simplistic, but for the purpose of fatigue and energy management, we need to emphasise the obvious.

When physical energy runs low, the payback results in exacerbated physical symptoms affecting your body. These may include swollen glands, sore throat, mouth ulcers, painful muscles, aching joints, heavy limbs, breathlessness, irregular body temperature control, hypersensitivities, digestive difficulties and disrupted sleep.

Here are some examples of physical energy activities:

- Coughing
- Turning in bed
- Sitting up in bed
- Standing from sitting
- Walking
- Showering
- Brushing teeth
- Combing hair
- Shaving
- Climbing the stairs
- Preparing food
- Eating food

- Tidying and cleaning
- Gardening
- Lifting and carrying
- Standing in a queue
- DIY
- Travelling.

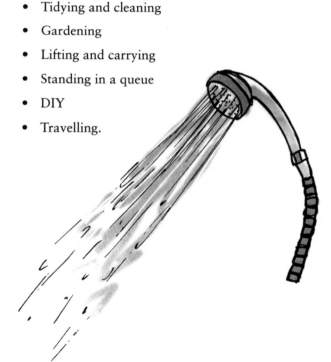

Now consider your situation. Which physical activities would you add to this list? Which would you remove?

Categorise each activity according to how costly it is for you. This is a subjective measure, which will be different for each person and may vary from day to day. Mark on your list:

- *High-energy activities:* these take a lot of energy, leaving you exhausted.

- *Medium-energy activities:* these are manageable but tiring.

- *Low-energy activities:* these can be completed with little effect.

Be aware over the coming days of your physical activities. Also, the amount of daily energy you spend on the different activities.

You know your body best.
Japanese proverb

TIP 41: CONSIDER COGNITIVE ENERGY

Cognitive energy is used for any activity with your mind.

When cognitive energy runs low, the payback results in exacerbated symptoms affecting your cognitive function. These may include brain fog, difficulties with memory, concentration, information processing, sequencing and word finding, sensory overload, headaches and dizziness.

Here are some examples of cognitive energy activities:

- Reading
- Writing
- Thinking
- Speaking
- Computer use
- Telephone use
- Finances
- Processing letters
- Mental maths
- Following instructions – verbal or written

- Problem-solving
- Answering questions
- Organising papers or tasks
- Recalling familiar information.

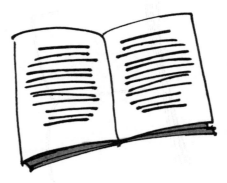

Now consider your situation. Which cognitive activities would you add to this list? Which would you remove?

Categorise each activity according to how costly it is for you. This is a subjective measure, which will be different for each person and may vary from day to day. Mark on your list:

- *High-energy activities:* these take a lot of energy, leaving you exhausted.

- *Medium-energy activities:* these are manageable but tiring.

- *Low-energy activities:* these can be completed with little effect.

Be aware over the coming days of your cognitive activities. Also, the amount of daily energy you spend on the different activities.

> You cannot see the brain on the forehead
> German proverb

TIP 42: CONSIDER SOCIAL/EMOTIONAL ENERGY

Social/emotional energy is used for any social/emotional activity.

When social/emotional energy runs low, the payback results in exacerbated symptoms and emotions affecting your energy and wellbeing. These may include less tolerance, impatience, tearfulness, feeling low, volatility, increased stress and anxiety, poor sleep, headaches, brain fog and an increase in physical symptoms.

Here are some examples of social/emotional energy activities:

- Talking and listening
- Being with other people in any setting
- All forms of social media
- Emails
- Phone calls
- Texting
- Shopping
- Public transport
- Relationship difficulties
- Conflicts and arguments
- Concern and worries
- Caring responsibilities
- Family life
- Work
- School/college/university
- Activities with friends.

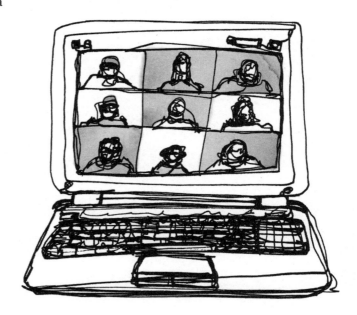

Now consider your situation. Which social/emotional activities would you add to this list? Which would you remove?

Categorise each activity according to how costly it is for you. This is a subjective measure, which will be different for each person and may vary from day to day. Mark on your list:

- *High-energy activities:* these take a lot of energy, leaving you exhausted.

- *Medium-energy activities:* these are manageable but tiring.

- *Low-energy activities:* these can be completed with little effect.

Be aware over the coming days of your social/emotional activities. Also, the amount of daily energy you spend on the different activities.

To be willing is only half the task.
Armenian proverb

TIP 43: CONSIDER DIFFERENT TIMES OF THE DAY

With regard to different times of the day, it is worth considering the following questions:

> 1. *When is your best time of the day?*

Why ask this?

People often have a natural tendency to either be a 'morning' person or an 'evening' person – either a 'morning lark' or an 'evening owl'. In other words, they are more alert and function better at certain points in the day. Perhaps you have experienced that this has changed completely since becoming ill? People affected by chronic fatigue frequently report that mornings are their worst time of the day and early evening is often the slightly better time of the day.

Knowing this is useful because:

> You may consider switching some activities to different times in the day to balance your energy supply and demand. Examples may be: washing your hair, preparing food for the next day or making necessary phone calls in the early evening, rather than the morning.

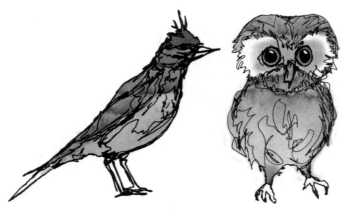

A LARK OR AN OWL?

2. Which time periods during the day demand most of your energy?

Why ask this?

Identifying the most demanding times of your day will enable you to plan, prepare and anticipate as far as you are able. Planning and preparation are very useful tools in managing decreased energy levels – it is like being your own friend and helper to your future self.

Knowing this is useful because:

You may consider keeping some time before and after these periods completely free. Avoid multi-tasking or arranging anything else during those time slots. Consider making some preparations at other times in the day to lighten the load. Examples may be: packing a work/school bag the night before, writing a shopping list the day before, preparing an evening meal in small chunks throughout the day or taking a shower the night before.

In the evening one may praise the day.
German proverb

TIP 44: CONSIDER DIFFERENT ENVIRONMENTS AND CONTEXTS

With regard to different environments, or contexts, it is worth considering the following questions:

> **1. *What are the most challenging environments for your energy levels?***

Why ask this?

Fatigue affects everyone in different ways. For some people being in a social context, needing to make conversation, listening to others and being aware of background noise can be more challenging than being in a cognitively demanding context such as an exam or test, or filling out a form. For others, a physically demanding environment, such as climbing stairs, having to stand, walking long distances and having nowhere to sit may be the more challenging environment. Becoming aware of the sensory effects on you personally of certain environments, such as bright lights, dark rooms, strong smells, noises and temperatures, can be enlightening and also empowering.

Knowing this is useful because:

> It is useful to identify the larger factors that influence your energy levels rather than thinking it is only your body or current level of capacity. It helps with planning and anticipating events in your day.

> **2. *How much energy does this environment, or context, cost me – High, medium or low?***

Why ask this?

> Frequently people may consider the energy demand of an activity but fail to

consider the environment or context. Sometimes, this takes more energy than the activity, as the following examples show.

Having a coffee with a friend:

a.   on a quiet park bench, a few metres from the car.

b.   in a noisy crowded shopping precinct with strong lighting, a long walk away from the car park.

Taking a short walk:

a.   on a dry flat path in good weather.

b.   on a sloping muddy path in the rain.

Knowing this is useful because:

It helps to plan and anticipate events in your day. It enables you to make wise choices for your health. You can still engage in more demanding environments, but having the foreknowledge allows you to plan more time and to pace the activity, thus remaining within healthy limits.

> Little by little the bird makes its nest.
> French proverb

TIP 45: CONSIDER DIFFERENT ACTIVITIES

Many years ago, when I was training to be an occupational therapist, we learnt how to analyse activities. I remember observing a local baker during his early morning shift. I noted every movement made and every process performed, just to make a loaf of bread. There were far too many for me to recall now.

> The point is that we often consider an activity, or task, as a whole rather than being aware of the multiple sections or chunks that make up the whole. Activity management is another term often used to describe pacing or fatigue management. Learning to break activities down into smaller parts is essential.

With regard to different activities, it is worth considering the following questions:

1. What are the various energy demands of this activity?

Why ask this?

> When you increase your awareness of the energy demands, it enables you to perform that activity in a healthy manner, including pacing and avoiding *boom and bust*. Doing this consistently will increase your capacity in the long term.

I spoke recently to a relative affected by long COVID fatigue. She had difficulty understanding why she was extremely fatigued following a very short walk that she had previously been able to complete with minimal after-effects. As we talked, a possible explanation became clearer. The first walk had been completed on her own; the second was with a friend. The first used physical energy; the second involved physical, social and cognitive energy.

Knowing this is useful because:

> It equips you for activity management and pacing. It helps you to plan, anticipate and balance your activities, which in turn helps you to move towards recovery.

2. How can I break this activity down into smaller parts?

Why ask this?

Basically, to manage your energy. Every activity can be broken down into smaller parts. It does not come naturally for us to operate this way, but if you can master it, you are halfway there.

To take an example, consider going shopping. Imagine that you can drive to the shops, purchase goods from two shops and drive home. The last time you achieved this, you were exhausted for the rest of the evening and did not sleep well. A healthier way to manage this activity might be to:

- prepare to go shopping and make a list
- sit for 2-3 minutes
- get into the car, without the radio on
- sit for 2-3 minutes
- drive to the shops and park nearby
- sit for 2-3 minutes
- go into one shop, observing if any chairs or benches are nearby
- sit for 2-3 minutes
- decide if you still want to go to the second shop
- go into the second shop, or not
- return to the car
- sit for 2-3 minutes
- drive home
- sit for 2-3 minutes before getting out of the car.

Knowing this is useful because:

This approach can be applied to everything you do that you have some control over. It takes longer to complete a task but will save time, in the long run, as you will not need as much time to recover.

He who begins much finishes little.
Bulgarian proverb

TIP 46: KEEP AN 'ENERGY COIN' IN RESERVE

Over the years I have heard many stories of people running out of energy just at the point when they most needed it.

Examples included running out of energy when:

- climbing the stairs at the end of the day
- getting ready for bed
- travelling home after being out
- trying to make sense when communicating with others
- trying to eat a meal
- taking an unexpected phone call
- just when getting to the main points during an interview or appointment.

Perhaps you have found yourself in similar situations?

Not only can these situations be frustrating and exhausting, but they often exacerbate your symptoms. Frequently they are at the end of your day and you resort to pushing through.

Using the metaphor of 'energy coins' (Tip 39), you are spending energy coins you do not have and find yourself overdrawn or bankrupt. You start the next day in deficit with depleted energy and fewer coins to spend that day.

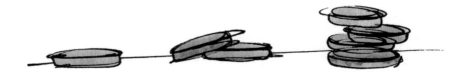

To avoid this, keep an 'energy coin' in reserve. Picture this coin in your pocket and your ability to draw upon it and spend it as and when it is needed.

Becoming skilled at this involves learning the importance of planning your day, pacing your activities, not pushing through; taking preventative rests (Tip 51) and recognising the energy costs of each of your everyday activities.

How can you start putting this into practice?

Don't let yesterday use up too much of today.
Native American proverb

TIP 47: DRINK MORE WATER, LIFE'S ENERGY DRINK

All of us in the Western world have the amazing resource of water easily within our reach and yet many of us do not drink enough of it each day.

> Even mild dehydration can have a significant impact on our daily health. If you experience cognitive symptoms, brain fog, headaches, dizziness and difficulties with memory and concentration, try drinking more water. Approximately 75% of our brain mass, more than any other parts of the body, consists of water.[20]

Fatigue, negative mood changes and nausea can also be signs of mild dehydration. Drinking more water can also prevent constipation and bladder infections.

Water also helps regulate our body temperature and maintain blood pressure, lubricates our joints, boosts our skin's health and supports our gums and oral health.

If you need to be convinced further about the benefits of drinking water, do an internet search. It will motivate you to drink more.

> Start today and drink more water

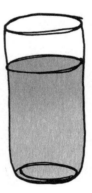

> Water is the strongest drink; it drives mills.
> German proverb

TIP 48: PUTTING ENERGY BACK IN

So far we have talked about all the things that will use energy and empty our piggy banks, but it is important to know that there are things we can do to add some coins to the bank too.

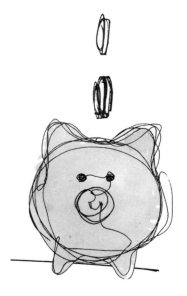

> What kinds of thing fill your daily energy piggy bank up?
>
> Where do you earn some of your energy coins for the day?

Here is what some people have told me:

a. Staying positive helps. A positive outlook helps you stay motivated and encouraged. The opposite is also true: discouragement drains your energy and motivation. This does not mean that you overlook the difficulties, but you make choices to position yourself in positivity.

b. Eating healthily. You need to put fuel into your body; calorific energy and hydration are essential (Tip 20, Tip 47).

c. Laughter and fun. Endorphins, the body's natural 'feel-good' hormones, are released with laughter. Choose to listen to music that makes you smile. Watch TV sitcoms that make you laugh. Watch some funny animal YouTube clips or read some jokes.

d. Relaxation and preventative rests (Tip 51).

e. Satisfaction in accomplishments. Celebrate every small achievement (Tip 35).

f. Hobbies and interests. So much of your daily energy is used in everyday necessary activities that it is difficult to have time for a hobby. Spending time enjoying an interest or hobby can feed your energy supply, simply because you are enjoying it ('Pause: Hobbies' on page 101).

Take some time now to consider your response.

What can you start doing to regularly put some daily coins back in your piggy bank?

A penny saved is twice earned.

German proverb

FOOD FOR THOUGHT

Comparing our body's energy usage to a battery is a familiar but useful metaphor. I worked alongside an amazing consultant for many years who often likened our energy to:

1. A car battery – If a car has been left unused for a few months, the battery would probably be flat. It would be flat from **underuse.** Some people can underdo, by being hesitant for fear of relapse, and stay well below their energy levels.

2. A torch battery – If a torch has been left on too long, the battery would probably

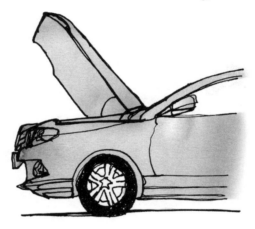

run flat. It would be flat from **overuse.** Some people may experience more energy one day and overextend themselves and crash the following day as per the *boom and bust* pattern.

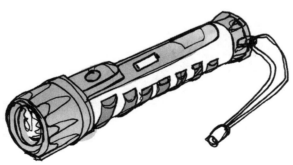

Neither underuse nor overuse is healthy and will only serve to perpetuate the fatigue. It is important to find ways to *balance* your energy – doing enough to keep your 'battery' topped up but not so much that you drain it completely.

PAUSE: SWITCHING

Practise *switching* your activities.

Switching activities is an effective pacing strategy to manage your energy.

- You can switch between different categories of activity: physical, cognitive and social/emotional.
- You can switch between different degrees of difficulty: high-, medium- and low-energy levels.
- You can switch between different environments: inside, outside, upstairs and downstairs.

I have seen this work in different ways for different people. Here are some examples:

1.

Get washed and dressed	Physical
Rest break	
Short phone call	Social/emotional
Rest break	
Computer search	Cognitive

2.

Morning	Afternoon	Evening
Cognitive	Physical	Social/emotional

How might you be able to practise switching?

MIND, BODY AND SOUL: ENERGY

Mind: What thoughts have you had as you read this chapter on Energy?

Other parts of the chapter you can let go of for now.

Body: What actions will you start putting into practice?

Soul: You may want to seek soul help with these changes. As explained in the book's Introduction, this section is from my perspective as a Christian, inviting God's help in the recovery process. You may have your own way of seeking soul help, so please do what you feel comfortable with.

Dear God, I ask you for help with my energy
and my recovery journey.
'He gives strength to the weary and increases the power
of the weak ... those who hope in the LORD will renew
their strength ... they will run and not grow weary,
they will walk and not faint.'[NIV]
Thank you, God.
Amen — may it be so.
Based upon Isaiah 40x[21]

CHAPTER 6

PACING AND ACTIVITY MANAGEMENT

'Pacing', 'activity management' and 'fatigue and energy management' are all names that describe, more or less, the same thing. Pacing is one of the main keys to unlock your road towards recovery.

> If fatigue management services could give you a medicine, or tablet, to treat the illness or symptoms you currently experience, the 'tablet' would be called 'pacing'.

So, what is pacing?

A friend of mine recently received a diagnosis of long COVID. She was told by her local doctor to 'pace yourself'. This is the correct advice, but she was unsure of what that meant in reality. Pacing can mean different things to different people. I wonder how you understand the phrase 'pace yourself'?

Some people think they need to slow down completely, rest as much as they can and put their feet up. Pacing certainly includes rest, but sadly, this is a frequent misinterpretation of pacing.

> Pacing is a way of balancing your energy and activities across time, be that an hour, a day, a week or a month. By pacing, you reduce the boom and bust pattern of fatigue, which then gives you a greater sense of control over your activities and the symptoms. It calms things down and gives you back more control, so that at last you can start to see your way through, rather than constantly being pushed around by horrendous symptoms and feelings of being out of control.

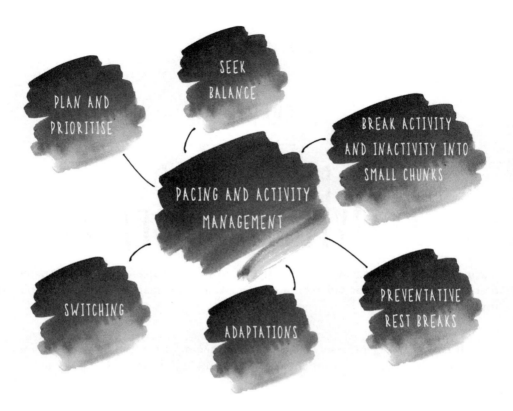

PLAN AND PRIORITISE

SEEK BALANCE

BREAK ACTIVITY AND INACTIVITY INTO SMALL CHUNKS

PACING AND ACTIVITY MANAGEMENT

SWITCHING

ADAPTATIONS

PREVENTATIVE REST BREAKS

There are different elements within pacing and activity management which enable you to learn what works best for you. Initially they involve seeking balance and operating within your limits, but with time, practice and some trial and error, you can change those limits in order gradually to increase your capacity.

TIP 49: UNDERSTAND THE GRAPHS

We considered in Tip 15 the 'boom and bust' pattern of fatigue. I wonder how aware you have become of that pattern in your daily activities?

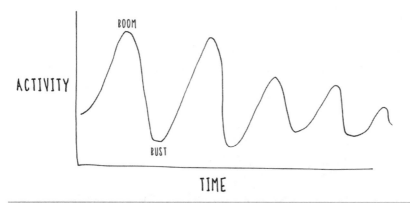

To establish balance, a baseline or a period of stability, we need to 'chop off' the top of the boom peaks and the bottom of the bust troughs on the graph. We need to learn how to hold ourselves back from doing too much (booming) and also encourage ourselves not to do too little (busting).

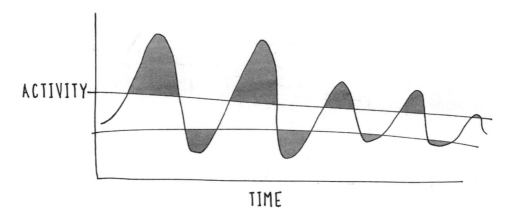

This can feel especially difficult when your level of activity is already significantly reduced by the fatigue, or conversely when you feel that you have crashed and have no choice but to rest. Within the capacity you have at the moment, it is important to recognise when to stop before you do too much (the boom, or overdoing things) and when to stop before you have to stop (the bust, or underdoing things).

> By doing this consistently, you start to maintain balance in your activity and energy levels. You are operating within your energy limits and not following the boom and bust pattern of fatigue.

When you are able to do this consistently, your capacity, and ability to do more, increases. This principle applies to all types of energy: physical, cognitive and social/emotional.

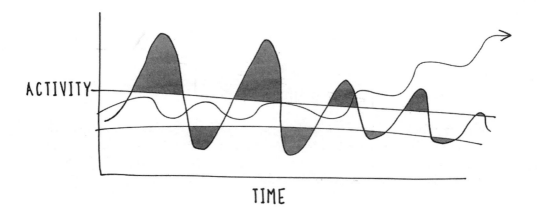

- Which parts of the graphs can you identify with?
- What may hinder you from 'chopping off' the top and bottom of the peaks and troughs?
- What may enable you to do this?

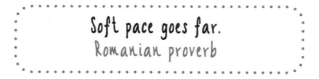

Soft pace goes far.
Romanian proverb

TIP 50: SEEK BALANCE — ESTABLISH A BASELINE

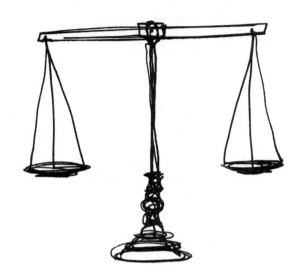

When you have learnt to stop before you do too much (the boom, or overdoing things) and also learnt to stop before you 'crash' and do too little (the bust or underdoing things), you will have found the right balance for your activity levels for this season. Sometimes this is referred to as 'establishing your baseline', which is illustrated by the grey section below.

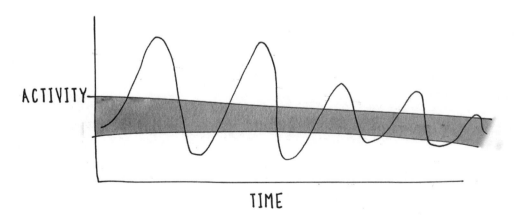

Your baseline activities are what you can do on a 'good' or a 'bad' day. They do not cause you to overdo or underdo things. On a 'good' day you may have to resist the urge to do more, especially when you are feeling able to. On a 'bad' day you may have to do certain baseline activities, regardless of how you feel, and resist the urge to be inactive. This enables you to stay healthy, balance your activity levels and stay within your baseline activities. This, over time, will result in a period of stability.

I have seen many relapses and setbacks occur during this period. When people feel able to do more on a 'good' day, they want to catch up on all the things they have been unable to do for so long. Unfortunately, they then pay the price for this in the following days, and sometimes weeks, which is known as post-exertional malaise (PEM).

The consequences are also true on a 'bad' day. When people decide to have a rest day or 'pyjama day', functioning below their baseline level and not doing their everyday activities, rather than restoration, the usual result is that they feel worse in the following days, and sometimes weeks.

On a 'good' day, break up the 'overdoing':

- Enjoy having a 'good' day and feeling somewhat lighter.
- Resist the urge to do more.

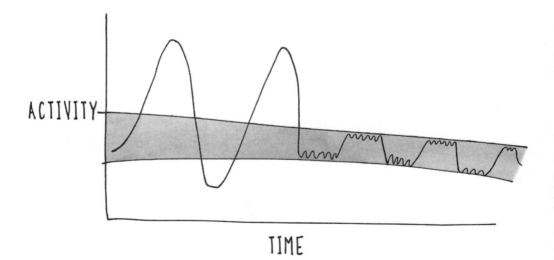

- Follow 'Pause: Take 5' on page 153 as often as you can throughout the day. This is the way to break up your overdoing.

- If you have at least 10 consecutive 'good' days, review your activity diary. It may be time to increase your baseline activity levels slightly (Tip 58).

On a 'bad' day, break up the 'underdoing':

- Be compassionate to yourself, and validate your frustrations. However, also try to remind and encourage yourself that the bad day will pass and that they are to be expected.

- Resist the urge to crash and underdo things.

- Keep to your basic balanced routine.

- Set a timer for 20-30 minutes and break up inactivity by moving, stretching and switching (see 'Pause: Star Stretch' on page 48 and 'Pause: Switching' on page 129).

- Plan in preventative rests (Tip 51) but avoid napping or oversleeping.

- If you have at least three consecutive 'bad' days, review your activity diary. It might be an indication that you need to decrease your baseline activity levels slightly (Tip 58).

> Who begins too much accomplishes little.
> German proverb

TIP 51: TAKE PREVENTATIVE RESTS

Preventative rests are planned short rest periods within the day. They are usually taken either late morning or early afternoon, but certainly before 4 pm. They are short – only 15-20 minutes' duration – and often at a similar time each day. Not everyone needs preventative rests, but if you find it hard to get through a day without falling asleep, then this tip is for you.

What is the difference between napping (which is discouraged) and preventative rests (which are encouraged)?

Daytime napping, or deep sleeping, is discouraged as it can be detrimental to recovery. This is because it usually mirrors the fatigue pattern of the *boom and bust* cycle and also affects your night-time sleeping quality and pattern. In other words, the fatigue is in charge and tells your body to nap or have a deep sleep. It is usually unplanned and comes from a place of exhaustion and necessity.

In contrast, a few preventative rests in a day can recharge your body's energy battery, prior to a potential crash in your energy supply. A preventative rest puts you in control and combats the b*oom and bust* cycle of fatigue.

How do I take a preventative rest?

To begin with, this involves trial and error to see what works best for you. Plan the timing of your preventative rest. This should occur after you have washed and dressed and had your breakfast, not before. Take your rest somewhere quiet and peaceful, with no distractions, where you can close your eyes. Some people prefer to lie down; others prefer to sit in a high-backed chair. Sitting up can certainly help if you are prone to falling asleep when you lie down. Close your eyes and relax for no more than 20 minutes.

If you discover that you are falling into a deep sleep, plan your rest at an earlier time in the day, or put in an additional rest. Also, look at the activities you were doing prior to the preventative rest: did you take enough pacing breaks during the activity?

Every few weeks, do not include preventative rests in your day. This will show if you still require them.

Nothing can exist long without occasional rest. Latin proverb

TIP 52: MAKE A PLAN

Are you naturally a planner?

Some people just love to plan, and others don't. Regardless of your natural preferences, planning is an important element in putting pacing into practice.

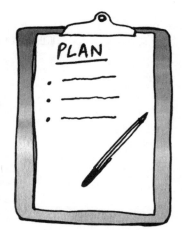

   Planning your activities, interspersed with pacing, enables you to get one step ahead of the fatigue and take back some control.

When you plan, include all your activities of daily living, such as getting washed and dressed and preparing your breakfast – basically, everything that you will spend your energy on. Keep in mind the tips and strategies you read about in Chapter 5.

What enables you in the planning process?

What hinders you in the planning process?

- Spend time organising the days of your week.

- Consider your best time of the day (Tip 43) and the environmental factors (Tip 44).

- Spread the activities throughout the week.

- Break the activities down into smaller parts (Tip 45).

- Switch around the activities from the different energy categories (physical, cognitive, social/emotional) and energy demands (high, medium, low) (Tips 40, 41, 42 and 'Pause: Switching' on page 129).

- Plan to avoid overexertion – for example, keep a basket at the bottom of the stairs for items to go upstairs, rather than going up and down unnecessarily.

- Don't over-plan, and keep some energy in reserve (Tip 46).
- Plan something that is energising (Tip 48).

Those who plan well, find love and truth.
Book of Proverbs[NIV]

TIP 53: PRIORITISE AND CHOOSE

Prioritise the activities and events that are important to you and your health. Prioritising *always* involves choice. You are making moment-by-moment choices as to what you spend your limited energy on, and what you do not.

Chronic illnesses often make you feel that your ability to choose has been taken from you. The fatigue has certainly stolen a lot of opportunities and options, in this season. However, each day you are making numerous decisions about your activities and health, without realising it.

For example, choosing to:

- take a break or not.

- push through or not.

- nap or take a preventative rest.

- eat junk food or eat healthily.

- relax before bedtime or stay longer on screens.

- get fresh air outside or stay indoors.

Recognising that you do have a choice over many small details can be empowering and liberating. Seek to recognise those small choices.

Prioritising certain activities is, and should be, a personal choice.

I have worked with people who have prioritised their appearance, choosing to spend extra time pacing their make-up and hair routine. Not only did it make them feel better, but it gave them a sense of wellbeing and achievement. I have worked with other people who did not prioritise their appearance, choosing to change into the same relaxed clothes and use dry shampoo for a few days so that they had energy for other things and less laundry to do. Both decisions worked perfectly for those individuals.

Spend a few moments considering what some of your priorities are.

> Health is an asset
> without equal.
> Basque proverb

PRIORITIES
1. HEALTH ✓
2. Social life
3. Work
4. House
5. Other demands

TIP 54: TRY ADAPTATIONS

Coping with limited energy for this season involves pacing and managing your activities.

> One useful way to manage your activities is to consider adaptations. This usually involves problem-solving and considering the most efficient method for any given task.
>
> By prioritising your energy for the things that are important to you, as in Tip 53, and using adaptations for other tasks, you use less energy. As well as environmental adaptations, it can also include such things as time and demands.

Here are a few examples of adaptations:

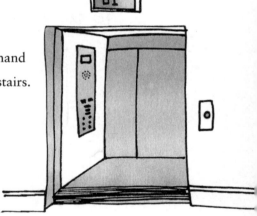

- Shower stools, kitchen stools, grab rails
- Online shopping and delivery
- Clearing clutter and keeping essential items to hand
- When out, using lifts or escalators rather than stairs.
- Having a parking pass
- Temporary wheelchair for longer trips out
- Keeping a basket at the top and bottom of the stairs to avoid unnecessary trips
- Time-saving appliances – dishwasher, tumble dryer
- Using coloured notes to remind yourself of important points
- Colour-coding important documents
- Alarm clock and timer
- Lighter bags
- Keeping a cushion and blanket in the car for taking a preventative rest
- Reducing work/college/school hours
- Reducing demands from responsibilities and people

- Adopting more sedentary hobbies for a while

- Reducing the length of social contact times for this season

- If finances permit, consider paying for a cleaner.

Most adaptations are usually for a season rather than permanent. I would not usually advocate any permanent environmental adaptations (such as stair lifts or ground-floor extensions) unless in exceptional circumstances, as this implies permanent disability rather than recovery.

Consider your own situation.

- Can you think of any useful adaptations that might save your energy for this season?

- What might enable you to start making those adaptations?

You cannot drive straight on a twisted lane.
Russian proverb

TIP 55: PACING EXAMPLE — PHYSICAL

PLAN AND PRIORITISE

IS THIS A PRIORITY TODAY?

WHEN IS THE BEST TIME OF DAY?

WHAT IS THE MOST ENERGY-EFFICIENT WAY TO SHOP?

PACING

WRITE A SHOPPING LIST. SIT FOR A FEW MINS.

TRAVEL TO SHOPS. SIT FOR A FEW MINS.

GO TO ONE SHOP. SIT FOR A FEW MINS.

GO TO ANOTHER SHOP. SIT FOR A FEW MINS.

GO TO TRANSPORT. SIT FOR A FEW MINS.

TRAVEL HOME. SIT FOR A FEW MINS.

UNPACK SHOPPING. SIT FOR A FEW MINS.

SHOPPING

ADAPTING

ONLINE SHOPPING.

SHOPPING TROLLEY OR USE A SMALLER BAG.

SHORTER TIME SHOPPING. LIMIT HOW MANY SHOPS.

PROXIMITY OF SHOPS. NEARBY?

CONSIDER ENVIRONMENT OF SHOPS: CHAIRS TO SIT DOWN, NOISE, CROWDS, SENSORY OVERLOAD, HELPFULNESS OF STAFF.

CONSIDER TRANSPORT: DRIVE, PUBLIC TRANSPORT, TAXI OR LIFT?

DELEGATE.

NOTES

DIFFERENTIATE ESSENTIAL SHOPPING SUCH AS FOOD AND HOUSEHOLD ESSENTIALS FROM ADDITIONAL SHOPPING. ITEMS SUCH AS GIFTS, EXTRA CLOTHES, COSMETICS, EQUIPMENT, GADGETS.

IF YOU ENJOY ADDITIONAL SHOPPING, GO ONLINE FOR ESSENTIAL SHOPPING AND USE YOUR ENERGY WITH PACING FOR SHORT ADDITIONAL SHOPPING TRIPS.

TIP 56: PACING EXAMPLE – COGNITIVE

PLAN AND PRIORITISE

WHEN DOES THIS NEED TO BE DONE BY?

WHEN IS THE BEST TIME OF DAY?

WHERE IS THE MOST DISTRACTION-FREE ENVIRONMENT? CLEAR CLUTTER, PHONES, NOISE, ETC.

WHAT IS MY REALISTIC PLAN OVER THE COMING DAYS OR WEEKS?

HOW CAN I SPREAD THIS OUT INTO HEALTHY CHUNKS OF ACTIVITY?

PACING

WORK FOR 10-15 MINS. NO MORE THAN 20, DEPENDING ON YOUR ABILITY.

STAND UP AND MOVE AWAY. BE IN A DIFFERENT ENVIRONMENT OR ROOM. STRETCH, WALK AND GET SOME FRESH AIR.

COME BACK AND WORK ANOTHER 10-15 MINS.

STAND UP AND MOVE AWAY. MAYBE DO SOME DIAPHRAGM BREATHING. SEE "PAUSE" IN CHAPTER 7.

COMBINE TAKING BREAKS WITH SWITCHING. SEE "PAUSE" IN CHAPTER 5. THIS IS PARTICULARLY EFFECTIVE WITH COGNITIVE ACTIVITIES.

STUDYING PAPERWORK COMPUTER WORK

ADAPTING

SOME PEOPLE HAVE FOUND ADAPTIVE TECHNOLOGY USEFUL SUCH AS VOICE-ACTIVATED DICTATION, TALKING BOOKS, ETC.

PHOTOCOPYING LECTURE OR CLASS NOTES RATHER THAN TAKING THEM YOURSELF.

IF POSSIBILE, DELEGATE HOUSEHOLD ADMIN. LIKE PAYING BILLS, ETC. RATHER THAN NEGLECTING OR STRUGGLING.

CLEAR YOUR ENVIRONMENT. SEEK TO BE FREE OF NOISE AND DISTRATION, NATURAL LIGHT, COMFORTABLE SEATING.

NOTES

REMEMBER, DOING 5 MINUTES IS BETTER THAN DOING NOTHING.

OFTEN, COGNITIVE DIFFICULTIES CAN BE FRIGHTENING, FRUSTRATING AND CONFIDENCE-KNOCKING. SEE BRAIN FOG TIP 87.

DRINK MORE WATER. TIP 47.

AVOID COMPARING YOUR CURRENT ABILITY WITH HOW IT USED TO BE AS THIS OFTEN LEADS TO FRUSTRATION AND SELF-CONDEMNATION. PRACTISE TIP 9.

SLEEP, ANXIETY, FATIGUE, DIET AND EXERCISE ALL HAVE A PROFOUND EFFECT ON COGNITIVE ABILITY.

TIP 57: PACING EXAMPLE – SOCIAL/EMOTIONAL

PLAN AND PRIORITISE

IF IT IS WITHIN YOUR CONTROL, PLAN THE MOST SUITABLE TIME OF DAY AND ENVIRONMENT.

BE ASSERTIVE WITH YOUR NEEDS "I CAN JOIN YOU FOR... BUT NOT FOR..."

ALLOW PLENTY OF TIME BEFORE AND AFTER THE EVENT.

INCLUDE ADDITIONAL PREVENTATIVE RESTS IN THE DAY BEFORE AND AFTER. SEE TIP 51.

PACING

TAKE REGULAR BATHROOM OR FRESH AIR BREAKS. SIT AND DON'T THINK FOR 5 MINS.

IF A LARGER SOCIAL EVENT, PRACTISE SWITCHING BY STANDING, SWOPPING SEATS AND DIFFERENT ROOMS.

TRY AND KEEP CONVERSATIONS BRIEF AND NOT INTENSE.

MEETING A FRIEND FOR A MEAL OR DRINK

ADAPTING

CONSIDER PERSONAL PREFERENCES FOR SOCIALISING WITHIN YOUR ENERGY LIMITS, WHICH STILL GIVE ENJOYABLE CONNECTIONS WITH OTHERS. FOR SOME THAT MAY BE ACTIVITIES SUCH AS :

...WATCHING TV

...PILATES OR RELAXATION

...COFFEE ON A PARK BENCH

...SHORT ZOOM CALL OR QUIZ

CONSIDER ENVIRONMENT. WHERE POSSIBLE CHOOSE PLACES THAT HAVE LESS SENSORY STIMULATION, AVOIDING LOUD MUSIC, CROWDS AND BRIGHT FLASHING LIGHTS.

NOTES

REMEMBER THE ENERGY COINS METAPHOR IN TIP 46. ALLOW ENOUGH ENERGY TO GET HOME.

BE AWARE THAT YOU MAY HAVE AN INCREASED SENSITIVITY TO ALCOHOL AND ITS EFFECTS.

LAUGHTER AND CONNECTION WITH OTHERS ARE ESSENTIAL FOR OUR HEALTH AND WELLBEING.

ENJOY! IF IT IS A STRUGGLE, PERSEVERE AND KEEP TRYING IN SMALL WAYS.

TIP 58: KNOW WHEN AND HOW TO INCREASE AND DECREASE ACTIVITY

Please do not take this tip in isolation until you have learnt to reflect on your own situation or tried to apply pacing and activity management.

This has to be an individual person-centred reflective approach. I cannot give you a formula or a percentage. However, I can give you some guidelines or broad brushstrokes:

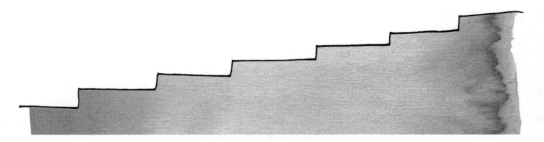

- For increasing and decreasing activity, always think in terms of slow small steps.

- Knowing when to increase is as important as knowing when to decrease.

- People tend to be either:
     a. too cautious to increase, due to fear of relapse, or
     b. too ambitious, increasing their activity too much, too quickly.

- You are likely to experience some discomfort with an increase and that is quite normal for a short while.

- However, if you are experiencing consistent exhaustion, and exacerbation of symptoms, for about three to five consecutive days, you have probably increased too much. You need to step back slightly and seek balance before trying again with a smaller increase.

- It is always trial and error, and thus important to try at the right time.

- As you become more experienced at reflecting, you will become aware of when you are ready to increase. Some people report restlessness, a feeling of boredom or a sense of more energy; others talk about having more space in their head, with new ideas and some sense of creative thinking.

- If you have at least 10 consecutive 'good' days, review your activity diary; it may be time to increase your baseline activities slightly.

- If you have at least three consecutive 'bad' days, review your activity diary; whilst making sure you are being careful not to underdo, (Tip 50), it may be time to decrease your baseline activities slightly.

- Be aware of other people's expectations and the pressures these cause – for example, some relatives, employers, educational establishments or medical professionals can sometimes encourage you to push beyond your limits.

- Take advice from your support team but remember that it is your body and your journey towards better health.

> You have to measure it to know if it is too long or too short.
> Korean proverb

FOOD FOR THOUGHT

What is the difference that makes the difference?

This is a famous concept, based on the work of Gregory Bateson,[22] an English anthropologist. It is frequently used in the world of family therapy.

It is one of those concepts that is simple, and yet profound, in its multiple applications.

It certainly influenced the way I worked as a therapist. In a therapy session, I would often introduce a '*difference*' - perhaps a suggested change someone could consider making, or a new perspective, or a new way of thinking.

If that difference was too big, it would usually be rejected.
It that difference was too small, it would usually be ineffective.

The same can be true regarding pacing applied to your varied everyday situations. Too big a difference and you may give up. Too small a difference and it will effect little change.

Consider for a moment:

What are some of the differences that may make the difference in your situation?

PAUSE: TAKE 5

Think of an activity that you are hoping to do today or tomorrow.

It is important to choose an activity that is within your current abilities – one that you have done recently.

It could be an activity of daily living, such as taking a shower, doing some laundry, cooking a meal, paying bills online or tidying up.

It could be a social activity, such as talking to someone on the phone, communicating on social media or meeting someone in person.

It could be a physical activity, such as going for a short walk, driving the car or going shopping.

It could be a cognitive activity such as reading, writing, thinking or planning.

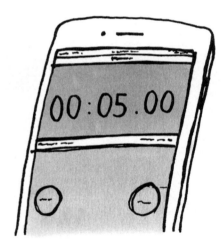

Set a timer for 5 minutes.*

Start the activity, keeping to your usual speed and style, but only do it for 5 minutes. Then STOP.

If you are able to, move away from the activity. Do nothing for 5 minutes.

Continue with the activity for 5 more minutes. Then STOP.

If you are able to, move away from the activity. Do nothing for 5 minutes.

Continue with the activity for 5 more minutes. Then STOP.

If you are able to, move away from the activity. Do nothing for 5 minutes.

You have just spent 15 minutes in activity and 15 minutes at rest.

The aim of breaking up this activity with rest periods is not to 'crash' and be exhausted at the end.

Notice how you feel after Take 5.

Try this with a variety of activities in the coming days.

---

* This activity can be changed to 2-3 minutes of activity if 5 minutes is too much

MIND, BODY AND SOUL: PACING AND ACTIVITY MANAGEMENT

Mind: What were your thoughts as you read this chapter on Pacing and activity management?

Other parts of the chapter you can let go of for now.

Body: What actions will you start putting into practice?

Soul: You may want to seek soul help with these changes. As explained in the book's Introduction, this section is from my perpective as a Christian, inviting God's help in the recovery process. You may have your own way of seeking soul help, so please do what you feel comfortable with.

Dear God, I ask you for help with pacing and activity management and my recovery journey.
'Trust in the LORD with all your heart and lean not on your own understanding ...
This will bring health to your body and nourishment to your bones.'[NIV]
Thank you, God.
Amen — may it be so.
Based upon Proverbs 3[23]

CHAPTER 7

MINDSET – ANXIETY

When chronic fatigue affects your health and interrupts your normal life, it brings with it a lot of uncertainty. Often there are many unanswered questions about your health, your ability to function and your future:

- How long will this go on?
- When will my capacity increase?
- What if I can't manage at work?
- When will I be able to … ?
- What if they don't understand?
- What if there is permanent damage?
- What will they think of me?

These concerns are not easily answered or solved. The ability to live with uncertainty, and the many 'What if?' questions, varies from person to person, day to day and circumstance to circumstance.

When uncertainty abounds, all too often anxieties rush in. They steal your peace by telling you all the things that could possibly go wrong. Before you know it, you are more exhausted from overthinking and less certain about the road ahead.

> Anxiety, stress, cares and worries (I have used the umbrella term of 'anxiety' for this chapter) are usually present with any chronic illness. One of the confusing factors with anxiety and chronic fatigue is that they share similar symptoms, such as unrefreshing sleep, exhaustion, pain, tension, altered appetite and digestion, headaches and memory and concentration difficulties. However, their management can be different.

Anxiety can start as a secondary issue to the chronic fatigue, but I have frequently seen this tip over to become the more dominant primary issue, which can prolong the fatigue and limit the ability to recover.

So how do we deal with anxiety?

Suppressing or ignoring anxiety can lead to more physical symptoms. Conversely, focusing too much on anxious thoughts can also lead to unhealthy symptoms. One of the key elements in dealing with anxiety is to acknowledge it and learn simple ways to manage it.

Whether you are highly experienced at managing personal anxieties or this is new for you, this chapter is applicable to everyone. Taking simple steps today to recognise and manage anxiety is necessary in order to focus your available energy on getting better.

TIP 59: ANXIETY CAN BE INFECTIOUS

We often think of laughter as being infectious. It is almost impossible not to join in, even if we do not know what the laughter is about. We often do not realise that anxiety is also infectious, but without the fun.

> If you are in an environment of anxiety and fear, you are more likely to become more anxious. Have you ever noticed how you can *'catch'* anxiety from other people – a bit like catching a cold? Have you ever walked into a room and sensed anxiety, almost as if it is in the atmosphere?

Let me give you an example:

I do not like going to the dentist. I often feel nervous. Prior to going, I clean my teeth well, go to the toilet a few times and feel slightly sick in my stomach. Yet I choose to go. When I arrive, either of these scenarios may await me:

Waiting room 1:

- Calming but loud music
- A small child screaming and the mother getting impatient at the long wait
- A man, sitting holding his face in pain, catches my eye and raises his eyebrows in despair
- Staff, rushing in and out, looking busy and overworked.

Waiting room 2:

- Calming, quiet music
- Pleasant magazines to distract me
- One of the receptionists calls me by my name. It reassures me that the staff know what they are doing and that things are under control
- I am told how long I will have to wait for my appointment.

Which atmosphere would you prefer? I have sat in both and I know which caused my anxiety levels to soar.

I have worked with many families where fear and anxiety have had a dominating presence in their lives and homes. This has affected their ability to function well and thrive. When working with families, to manage anxiety it is always amazing to witness how, when one person makes small positive changes, this can affect the whole family.

- Recognise the influence that you and others have on the atmosphere.

- Choose wisely which atmosphere you want to be in.

- Take note of how the media affects you – music, TV, social media – as sad news can fuel fear and anxiety.

Better to eat bread in peace, than cake amid turmoil.
Slovak proverb

TIP 60: RECOGNISE THE PHYSICAL SIGNS OF ANXIETY

When our bodies come under threat or stress, the hormones adrenaline and cortisol are triggered. These hormones cause our heart to beat faster and divert our blood to where it is needed most. This causes various symptoms in our body illustrated below. We are prepared for action and this is known as the 'fight, flight or freeze' response.

Simply put, if you were living in Stone Age days and a bear suddenly appeared, what would your response be? Your body would immediately, without delay, jump into action. You would either attack the bear (fight) or run away as fast as you could (flight). Whatever response you chose, your hormones would have done an amazing job of preparing your body for action and keeping you safe. There is also the freeze response where you are completely paralysed and do nothing; if there is no hope of escape or fighting back, not

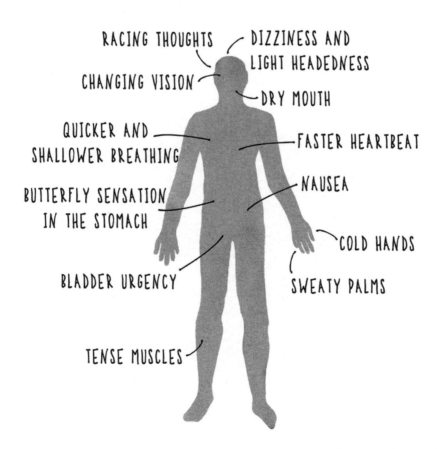

RACING THOUGHTS

DIZZINESS AND LIGHT HEADEDNESS

CHANGING VISION

DRY MOUTH

QUICKER AND SHALLOWER BREATHING

FASTER HEARTBEAT

NAUSEA

BUTTERFLY SENSATION IN THE STOMACH

COLD HANDS

BLADDER URGENCY

SWEATY PALMS

TENSE MUSCLES

being noticed may be the best option. After the threat had gone, your body and muscles would have then relaxed.

> Anxiety has a way of keeping us in that place of 'fight, flight or freeze'. Our bodies can get exhausted and unable to relax after a heightened sense of alert and possible threat.

- In your body, which physical signs of anxiety do you notice first?
- Which do you notice next?
- Which physical signs of anxiety are similar to chronic fatigue symptoms?

> Anxiety weighs down the heart.
> Book of Proverbs[NIV]

TIP 61: RECOGNISE THE ANXIOUS BEHAVIOURS YOU DISPLAY

Anxiety tends to creep towards us and, before we know it, can leave us feeling overwhelmed. We tend to focus on our emotions and feelings, rather than our actions and behaviours.

> Strong emotions always lead to behaviour; we either *do* or *do not do* something as a result. Recognising our behavioural patterns can help us identify anxiety quickly, before it has time to build up. This can also help reveal potential solutions and ways forward.

To give you a simple example, the early behaviours I frequently display when I start to feel anxious are:

- I get restless but try to sit still and appear calm.
- I then move around a lot, either pacing up and down or tidying somewhere. I tend to be moving and doing.
- I write lists of what I need to do and often check my diary.
- My immediate response to, 'How are you?' is, 'I am fine', and I usually do not ask for help at this stage.
- I usually go to the toilet and feel thirsty.
- I sigh a lot – a weary sigh.
- I often become warm and flushed.

> Often, we ignore early behavioural signs and do not acknowledge the underlying anxiety. Being aware, and naming what you are experiencing, enables you to appreciate how you are feeling and some of that is okay. At other times, being aware enables you to employ strategies promptly to prevent the anxiety from escalating.

- When you are experiencing anxiety, what do you do?
- What patterns of behaviour do you display?

- Are you able to spot these early in the process?

> Worrying is like sitting in a rocking chair. It gives you something to do but it doesn't get you anywhere.
> English proverb

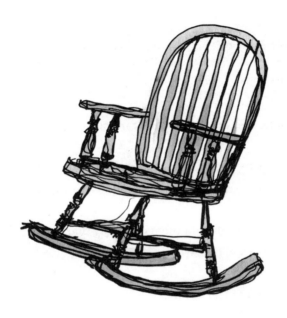

TIP 62: NOTE YOUR THOUGHTS AND THEIR EFFECTS

Your thoughts are powerful and affect your emotions, behaviour and physical reactions, as this illustration shows.

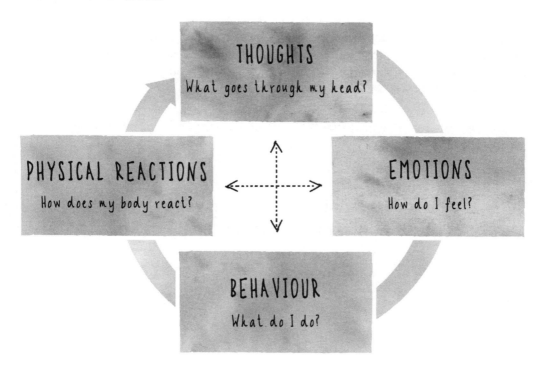

When you experience anxiety, often your thoughts can race. You may be overthinking – trying to make sense of your situation or seeking reassurance and relief from the current discomfort. It can be exhausting.

> If you notice what is going through your mind, you can try to 'catch' your thoughts. Trying not to think about something does not work, but becoming aware of your thoughts and replacing regular unhelpful thoughts or punitive language with alternative thoughts has proved to help countless people.

This is similar to Tip 9 where you practised reframing descriptions of yourself. Thoughts such as:

- 'Not sure I will cope' could be, 'It may be difficult – but I could try'.

- 'I will be ill throughout' could be, 'I am unsure how my body may react'.

- 'They will think I am stupid' could be, 'I feel somewhat self-conscious but I will focus on others'.

- 'What if I have a relapse from doing too much?' could be, 'If I have a dip it is okay and I will manage'.

Also, practise changing the words 'should' and 'must' to 'could and 'might'.

Recognising the power of your thoughts and their effect on your feelings, emotions, behaviour and physical reactions can be liberating. This awareness enables you to have some choice and control over your thoughts, however small.

> Recognising the power of your thoughts allows you to reframe them and make healthier choices.

Thinking well is wise; planning well is wiser; but doing well is the wisest.

Iranian proverb

TIP 63: SPOT AVOIDANCE

As we have already discussed, one of our body's main strategies for dealing with threatening situations is the 'fight, flight or freeze' response. This can cause us to avoid certain events and situations that provoke uncomfortable feelings (Tip 60).

We all welcome avoidance of danger which keeps us safe. However, avoidance left unchecked can reduce our opportunities and cause us to miss out on many enriching activities for our rehabilitation and recovery.

When a situation arises, and various symptoms of anxiety are triggered, we have a choice to either:

    a. take steps forward into that situation, or

    b. avoid it.

Many people affected by chronic fatigue have told me, in retrospect, that avoidance has often happened as a result of their cancelling or backing out of situations due to 'illness'. Later they have become aware of fears and anxieties, often related to concerns about coping, potential setbacks and feeling vulnerable.

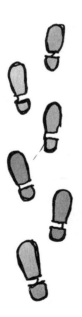

Avoidance gives immediate relief. The situation, and the demands that came with it, has gone and, as a result, the symptoms have settled down. However, this relief is only short-term. Procrastination is also a type of avoidance.

The longer-term consequence of avoidance is that future similar situations become even harder and your comfort zone gradually becomes reduced.

- Are you able to spot avoidance?

- What situations do you avoid?

- Can you distinguish between fatigue and anxiety?

- When anxiety is present, what may help you to choose to take steps forward, rather than avoidance?

> The toad that wanted to avoid the rain fell in the water.
> African proverb

TIP 64: KEEP YOUR HEALTH CONCERNS IN CHECK

With most chronic illnesses that involve multiple symptoms, there have usually been medical investigations (e.g. blood tests) to eliminate other causes. This is when a diagnosis of CFS/ME or long COVID is likely to be given. It should be reassuring that the symptoms have been checked and nothing has been found, but it can often leave people wondering if something has been missed.

> There has been a lot of fear in our society about catching COVID-19. We have all had to practise being extra vigilant with regard to our behaviour and our bodily sensations. Do I have symptoms or not? This heightened awareness has been out of concern for our safety, and those around us, but it has certainly caused an increase in anxiety about health. It can be challenging to hold a balanced view.
>
> Being anxious and excessively focused on the symptoms can be exhausting. It often makes you feel worse, as the significance of each symptom tends to be amplified. This can cause a delay on your road to recovery. All the energy spent on researching your symptoms could be better used to take small positive actions towards your recovery.

Be aware and take steps if:

1. You are spending long periods of time online, checking 'Dr Google', researching symptoms, reading health-related social media sites, etc:

   - Try limiting the amount of time you spend online.

   - Take note if you are feeling reassured or more anxious after your research. Have a break from social media/online searches for a few days.

2. You are checking your body for particular symptoms frequently, thinking about them a lot, observing them, talking about them, and/or booking additional doctors' appointments. You are finding it hard to think about anything else.

   - Select some distraction activities and focus your attention and energy on these, such as watching TV, doing a puzzle or going for a short walk if able

   - If you need to get checked out by your local doctor whom you trust, do it once but avoid unnecessary appointments.

3. You are having regular unhelpful negative thoughts, such as, 'What if I have a brain tumour? I must have a brain tumour because ...'

   - Capture these regular thoughts and jot them down.

   - Consider what a more balanced or reasonable thought might be and jot that down too.

4. You are having regular, unhelpful negative, health-related images, perhaps from being in hospital or from other traumatic events. This is often your brain's way of trying to make sense of what occurred.

   - At that moment, distract your attention onto your immediate surroundings: what you can hear, what you can see, what you can feel, what you can smell, what you can taste.

Trying to suppress negative thoughts and feelings only makes you feel worse and usually does not work. Follow the tips above in order to avoid spending an excessive amount of your energy worrying about your health.

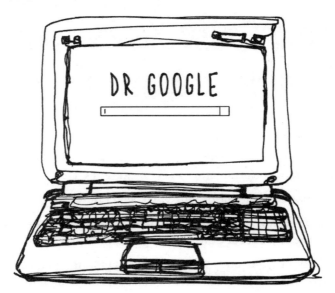

When a tiny toe is hurting, the whole body stoops
down to attend to it.
African proverb

TIP 65: KEEP ANY SOCIAL ANXIETIES IN CHECK

Chronic fatigue limits your social capacity. When you are not feeling well, it is normal to curtail social time with other people. Curtailing socialising for short periods has few ill effects. However, when the weeks turn into months, socialising again can, at times, become like a mountain to climb. As seen in Tip 18, social anxiety can become a more dominant issue than chronic fatigue if left unchecked.

The pandemic has only exacerbated this issue for us all, regardless of having chronic fatigue or not. Isolating, living through lockdowns and social distancing, have perhaps left us all experiencing some loneliness, which has knocked our social confidence. We all need to begin exercising our 'social muscle' again in an ever-changing society.

It is normal to experience some of the physical symptoms of anxiety, such as rapid heartbeat, light-headedness, sweating, blushing, difficulty speaking and sometimes shaking when we are attempting things again after a long time.

Take note if you are doing any of the following.

1. Cancelling social situations: This is avoidance (see Tip 63) and only exacerbates the situation and makes it harder for you next time. Try the following:

   - Keep fatigue in check before and after an event (Tip 57).

   - Take short pacing breaks if you can.

2. Worrying about social situations more than necessary; overthinking and considering all potential pitfalls. Try the following:

   - Limit thinking by having 'worry times' (Tip 66).

   - Think of something positive about this situation.

   - Get a support team to cheer you on from a distance (Tip 37).

3. Excessively focusing on yourself and your symptoms, worrying that you may embarrass yourself or that people will think badly of you. Try the following:

   - Do some relaxation breathing techniques prior to the event.

   - Slow down and pay extra attention to what is around you. Listen to what people say; look at their faces. What can you smell, touch, hear, see, taste? This will distract you from thinking about yourself and will help you to be fully present where you are.

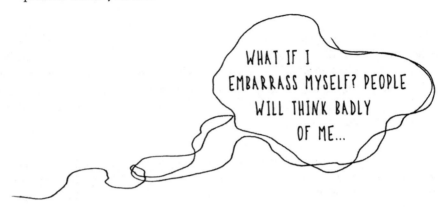

4. Experiencing excessive negative self-talk after an event, analysing and overthinking.

- Try and let it go. Be kind to yourself (Tip 38).
- Limit the time you spend thinking (Tip 66).
- Capture some of those familiar negative comments and positively reframe them (Tip 9).

When building up social activities, it is wise to start with people who are understanding and accommodating. Others, who don't understand your limited capacity, may have higher or more demanding expectations. If this is your experience, create some assertive sentences which express your needs in a comfortable manner, such as:

'I would love to spend a bit of time with you. I have been struggling with my energy levels recently due to long COVID. What I can do is ...[insert your limit here, e.g. come for a cup of tea for half an hour] and I also ask that we only meet if you are healthy.'

Worry often gives a small thing a big shadow.
Swedish proverb

TIP 66: HAVE A 'WORRY TIME'

If you find yourself thinking a lot about concerns or anxieties throughout the day or night, this Tip is for you.

Having a specific time set aside to worry can sound a little strange but this is a technique that many people have found to be useful. Often the worries and anxieties can dominate if left unchecked. Keep a list and jot down concerns as they crop up through the day, but delay thinking about them until the prearranged 'worry time'.

> Keeping your thinking about these concerns confined to this allotted time helps put you back in control of your thoughts. It also guards the rest of your day's time and energy, allowing you to spend it on more healthy pursuits.

This practice often gives people a realisation that worries can be thought about briefly and do not require overthinking or an excessive amount of time.

- Set aside 15-20 minutes each day, but not late in the evening before sleep.
- At the start of the week, plan daily time slots for the 'worry time'.
- Find somewhere quiet and distraction-free to do this.
- Look at the list of worries you took note of during the day. Some may now be resolved, some you may be able to problem-solve and others may need to stay on the list for now.
- Distinguish between worries that are out of your control and those that you can do something about.
- Schedule paced action today for the worries that you can do something about.

I have also seen this work well with parents and young people when it has been a joint decision to have a 'worry time'.

> Every little yielding to anxiety is a step away from the natural heart of man.
> Japanese proverb

TIP 67: GROW BRAVERY

> Managing, and overcoming, anxiety involves reducing time spent *thinking* about worries and increasing time spent *doing*. It is impossible just to *think* your way out of anxiety.
>
> **Brave people feel scared, but they do whatever it is they are scared of doing anyway.**

Bravery is finding the courage to take steps forward and do something now. It involves facing your fears and doing what needs to be done. Bravery steps into opportunities rather than avoiding them. It is necessary for journeying towards your preferred future.

How can you grow bravery?

- Do things in small chunks, one very small step at a time.

- Avoid overthinking (Tip 66). Try not to compare present achievements with past achievements.

- With any brave steps that you take, practise saying 'Well done' to yourself.

- Be aware of your feelings and fears. You can run away from them and miss out, or feel your feelings and do what you set out to do.

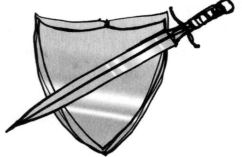

- Grow in your ability to tolerate uncertainty. Let go of some control; perhaps let someone else make a plan; try to be more spontaneous; reduce your tendency to overplan.

- Don't be fearful of failure. Toddlers learn to walk by repeatedly falling over; a lot of life's experiences include trial and error and it is part of the journey to recovery. Perfectionist tendencies often lead to high expectations of yourself; combined with chronic fatigue, this can attack your courage and leave you feeling far from brave.

- Expand your comfort zone. Challenge yourself little by little with the things that you are avoiding or feeling anxious about.

- How brave are you at present? From 0 (not very brave) to 10 (very brave) out of 10?

- What can you do to be one step braver?

Bravery is not the absence of fear;
it is action in the face of fear.
English proverb

TIP 68: FIND YOUR PEACE

We all try to find peace in different ways. What peace means, and may look like, to one person may appear and mean something very different to someone else. We may describe it differently, such as calm, relaxed, chilled, soothed, balanced, on an equilibrium, stress-free.

You may experience a certain amount of peace when you go on holiday. You are away from circumstances and events that normally bring stress and demands into your life. You tend to look after yourself and sleep, eat and relax better than in your normal life. We all know that holidays come to an end, and you cannot live your life always avoiding the stress and strain of everyday life, but you can seek to look after your health and wellbeing.

Sometimes you may need that 'in the moment' immediate peace to calm your nerves as you take a courageous step forward or prevent a panic attack. For some people that can be achieved by deep breathing, saying a prayer, taking a short break, focusing on nature and noticing the detail and effortlessness of it all, or talking to someone. Try to discover what helps you find your peace in those immediate situations, as it will enable you to take steps forward.

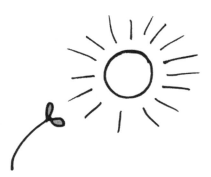

At other times, you may need to find your peace during life's ups and downs, and uncertainties. Avoid turning to substances such as alcohol or tobacco, as they are poor substitutes for peace. For some people, peace is relaxing in a bath, listening to a radio program or watching a sitcom. For others it is gardening, gentle stretching, mindfulness, meditation, cooking, knitting, reading, singing, praying, laughing or talking.

- In what ways do you experience peace?
- What may help you experience more peace?

A heart at peace gives life to the body.
Book of Proverbs[NIV]

FOOD FOR THOUGHT

Worrying is carrying tomorrow's load with today's strength — carrying two days at once.

Worrying doesn't empty tomorrow of its sorrow, it empties today of its strength.[24]

Corrie ten Boom, Ravensbrück concentration camp survivor

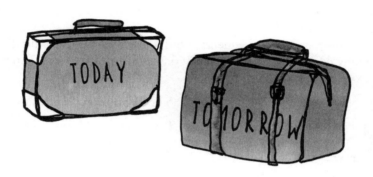

PAUSE: BREATHE FROM YOUR DIAPHRAGM

We often breathe from our upper chest which, when combined with poor posture, can result in not filling and emptying our lungs fully and also in neck and back pain. When we experience anxiety, our breath tends to be rapid and shallow and, if this pattern is constant, can lead to hyperventilation, panic attacks and further distress. Learning to counter this with deep, calm breathing is always beneficial.

Deep diaphragm breathing has many positive effects on our body and wellbeing. The vagus nerve is the longest cranial nerve in the body. Diaphragm breathing can stimulate this nerve to relax the body.[25] The *'fight, flight or freeze'* response is calmed, endorphins are released and the blood flow is increased.

Try practising deep breathing frequently until it becomes a more natural occurrence.

There are many different methods of doing this. Find one that you are comfortable with. Here is one example for you to try:

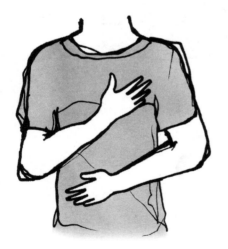

- Sit or lie down comfortably in a calm place.
- Place one hand on your stomach below your rib cage and the other on your upper chest.
- Relax and notice how you are breathing.
- Try and exhale for longer than normal.
- Breathe in slowly through your nose and feel your stomach rise and expand downwards.
- Exhale slowly through your mouth.
- Be aware of your hand on your chest, which should remain still.
- Repeat for five breaths.
- Start by doing this once a day and gradually build up to four to five times a day.

MIND, BODY AND SOUL: MINDSET — ANXIETY

Mind: What thoughts have you had as you have read this chapter on Anxiety?

Other parts of the chapter you can let go of for now.

Body: What actions will you start putting into practice?

Soul: You may want to seek soul help with these changes. As explained in the book's Introduction, this section is from my perspective as a Christian, inviting God's help in the recovery process. You may have your own way of seeking soul help, so please do what you feel comfortable with.

Dear God, I ask you for help with the anxiety
and my recovery journey.
'Cast all your anxiety on him because he cares for you.
'In every situation ... present your requests to God.
'And the peace of God, which transcends all understanding,
'will guard your hearts and your minds in Christ Jesus.'NIV
Thank you God.
Amen — may it be so.
Based upon 1 Peter 5 Philippians 4²⁶

CHAPTER 8

COMMUNITY AND RELATIONSHIPS

As the familiar saying goes, 'No man is an island'. We are all connected in some shape or form to other people. As you are fully aware, chronic fatigue affects you personally in relationships. It limits your capacity for socialising and relating to other people at present. As with all chronic illnesses, this not only affects you individually but all the people that you are connected to.

Those you are closest to, people you conduct everyday life with, are also adapting to the limitations of the chronic fatigue. For some of you, it is your immediate family. For others, it is friends and workmates, or a combination. These are your significant relationships: the people that you know and care about and the people who know and care about you. Roles and responsibilities shift and change; family dynamics often have to alter out of necessity due to the fatigue.

There are also the wider community relationships: people on the streets, in the shops, on public transport, in public and health services, with whom you would normally cross paths if you were able to go about your everyday life. This reciprocal interaction of smiling, making comments and general chit chat, with people you barely know, has a way of filling your emotional tank and giving a sense of belonging and contribution, more than you often realise. During the pandemic, we all experienced the loss of some of these wider community interactions and felt its effects. Energy is often kept for your close family and friends, so wider community socialising may have to be put on hold for a while.

Amongst all these changes, loyal family and friends do care. They often want to support and help you but sometimes do not know how. They are also going through their own process of adjustment and trying to make sense of the illness. Sometimes that can be expressed as anger towards you, maybe for the loss and limitations that the fatigue now places on them and on your relationship. It can also be expressed as having totally unrealistic goals and expectations for you, in an attempt to overcome the fatigue quickly. Sadly, the fatigue does not play by those rules and remains as that uninvited visitor in the relationship.

In therapy sessions, I have heard stories of wonderful support, understanding and care from relatives. I have also heard stories of frustrating or exhausting family dynamics – perhaps unasked-for advice, criticism, misunderstandings, unhelpful comments, judgements or too much unwanted attention, or arguments and conflicts. Frequently, when the time was taken gently to discuss what had occurred, different perspectives and *the intentions* behind the unwanted or annoying behaviours that had been expressed, it was nearly always clear that these behaviours arose out of love and concern. It never ceased to amaze me how clearer communication, greater understanding and/or simple tools could release such a flow of reciprocal care, love and support that those dynamics shifted to be healthier and more supportive.

In this chapter, we will concentrate mostly on the effects of the fatigue on close relationships, with useful tips.

TIP 69: CONSIDER INDEPENDENCE/DEPENDENCE

In our western societies, we highly value independence. We place a lot of emphasis on raising our children and adolescents to be independent young adults. We hope that they will be able to 'stand on their own two feet' and cope with the many challenges that life brings along their path. This independence often leads to our nuclear families being private and self-sufficient. At times, this can lead to loneliness, isolation and difficulty in asking for help or support, if needed.

In contrast, one of my dear Ugandan friends often quotes the phrase, 'It takes a village to raise a child'. She talks warmly of community involvement in family life. We often need each other more than we think.

> We may all vary with our values and views on personal independence, but one thing I am sure we will all agree upon is that chronic fatigue and illness affect our independence and relationships.

This fact was very telling when I worked with adolescents affected by chronic fatigue syndrome. Parents sacrificed much to care for their ill teenagers, and frequently had to cut back on work commitments and income to do so. They often had to act as an advocate for them with education and medical professionals and with extended family members. All of this was necessary due to the illness but was out of sync with the offspring's age and stage of life. This necessary caring role would often continue for some time. Then, as health returned and recovery gradually increased, the parents crucially had to adjust their role too.

> Stepping back from being a carer was essential for the young person to grow in independence. Occasionally this stepping-back stage proved to be more difficult and at times, when delayed, hindered progress by continuing the dependence. The same relational pattern can occur with couples too.

Loss of independence can be frustrating. For some, being the recipient of care can be hard. If you are able, try to acknowledge your feelings and emotions. At times, you may be taking this anger and frustration out on those closest to you.

- If you are able to, express gratitude to those who are assisting you.

- Always keep in mind that this is only for a season.

- Evaluate and adjust your roles as you start to recover.

> It is observed that, in a great endeavour, it is not enough for a person to depend solely on himself.
> Native American proverb

TIP 70: FAMILY

Family can mean different things to different people. For the purpose of this tip, I am referring to the people who are closest to you and perhaps live in the same home. Family members know you well. They often see you 24/7 and know you *'warts and all'*, as we say in the UK. They observe your ups and downs and they too are affected and confused by the fatigue.

> As you are all too aware, the fatigue affects each member of your household also. The whole family dynamic shifts to accommodate the fatigue. Issues I have frequently heard from families include:

'They don't understand': Sadly no one fully understands and we are all still trying to make sense of COVID-19 and chronic fatigue. Try to encourage them to read this book or look at some useful leaflets. Maybe ask them to accompany you to some medical appointments. Perhaps they understand more than you think and they may be trying to 'fix' the problem in their own particular way.

'They are always giving advice or correction': Often family members can be just as frustrated and angry about the fatigue and its effects as you are. Sometimes, in attempting to bring some order out of the uncertainty, they can fall into advice-giving mode in an attempt to solve and fix it. Instead of having the desired effect, this can leave you feeling isolated and unsupported. Take time to talk, maybe using the Holding something exercise (Tip 75 no 5). Encourage them to continue their support and regularly discuss together alternative support and family ways to deal with the fatigue.

'I am trying to keep strong and I don't want to be a burden': Often family want to support and help but do not always know how. You will at times need help and support (Tip 37) and that is okay for now and for this season (Tip 1). Families are often more resilient than we think. Be aware of carrying unnecessary guilt (Tip 82) or burdens or expecting too much of yourself. This only drains your energy and prolongs recovery. Active acceptance of the limitations of the current season is important for continued recovery (Tip 33).

'What about the rest of the family?': In larger families, this concern is often raised. When one member of the family has chronic fatigue, much attention and care is focused on that individual - adult or child. Frequently this care tends to fall predominantly on one adult. Younger children can observe that illness gets attention from that adult. Try to share and mix care-giving roles as much as possible. Delegate to grandparents, and good friends, in order that time and attention can also be given to healthy children.

'Everyone is dealing with it in their own way': This sounds quite normal. Everyone will be responding to the fatigue in their own way and no doubt all at different stages. They may each have their own anxieties and fears about your recovery. It is important to have healthy boundaries and not take on board other adults' emotions yourself. Younger children may require reassurance that you are okay.

Some families have found regular weekly checking-in times useful where they talk about positive or difficult issues as they arise. Other families just want to hang out together more. Communication and time to be together are key. You probably know your family and their needs better than anyone.

There is no place like home.
British proverb

TIP 71: BALANCING CARING RESPONSIBILITIES

> The majority of people affected by chronic fatigue are people with roles and responsibilities, commitments and a web of interwoven relationships.

Some of you reading this book will have responsibilities for caring for other people. They may be your own offspring – babies, toddlers, children, adolescents – or blended family responsibilities at certain times in the week. There may be someone with a disability, mental health condition or special needs within your household, or elderly dependent relatives who require your care and attention. You may have people to share that responsibility with, or you may be juggling their needs on your own.

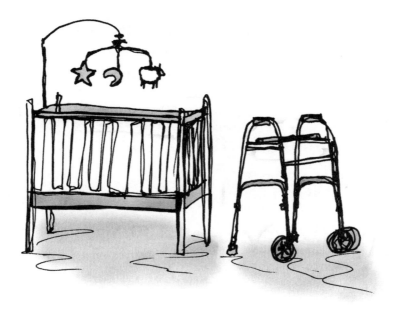

Most of these caring responsibilities are essential and some, such as for babies and children, would become a safeguarding issue if neglected. Some may not be as essential and could be cut back upon in order for you to prioritise your recovery (Tip 4, Tip 53). A UK survey of 8000 carers[27] discovered that 64% of them focused on the care needs of the person they cared for rather than their own.

For you to improve, your recovery journey needs to be a high priority.

- Evaluate your current caring responsibilities and see if you can protect time for yourself.

- Which tasks can or cannot be delegated?

- Consider who can step in to assist you or take on more responsibility.

- Plan and manage routines that work both for your needs and those you care for.

- Some things may need to be just 'good enough' in this season, and that is okay.

- Research if there are any supports, charities or services available locally.

I've got your back, you've got mine.
American proverb

TIP 72: INTIMATE SEXUAL RELATIONSHIPS

Healthy sex is a beautiful reciprocal intimate way of communicating love, tenderness and care between two consenting adults – both giving and receiving. Not all sex is healthy and, for many of us, sex can also have different meanings, connotations, memories, desires and effects.

If able to discuss sex, chronic fatigue sufferers frequently report frustrations and inadequacies due to a low sex drive and lack of energy. They think they are letting their partner down or putting unrealistic expectations upon themselves. I have also heard people say that sex highlighted their partner's lack of understanding about the fatigue, leaving them at times feeling isolated and sad.

Sex is a form of mild to moderate exercise. It requires physical and emotional energy and yet it can, at times, be truly energy-giving too. Physical touch and union can often nurture, comfort and feed our bodies and souls in ways that words cannot. Cardiac rehabilitation often compares the energy or fitness required for sexual intercourse to that of being able to walk up two flights of stairs without getting out of breath.[28] Everyone is different but sometimes it can be useful to have an objective measure like that.

Many long COVID and chronic fatigue sufferers struggle to 'spend' that much energy, as they often do not have it. It is important to be able to discuss your sexual relationship with your partner as early as you can so that it doesn't become a bigger issue than it needs to.

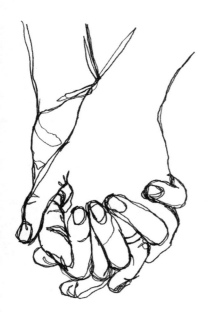

Try to discover ways that you both find comfortable and pleasurable within this season.

Some practical considerations include:

- Find new approaches to express affection and touch.

- 'Plan leisurely times to relax and be intimate. For some, this involves plenty of cuddles but not full sex; for others it may be little and often.

- Consider, if circumstances allow, changing the time of the day to when you have more energy.

- Have regular times when you can check in with each other and talk, allowing understanding and pleasure to grow.

- Be kind to yourself and your partner; it is an adjustment for both of you.

Kisses are the messengers of love.
Danish proverb

TIP 73: FRIENDS

Friendships can be invaluable during this season. Having friends that you can be yourself with, who accept you as you are despite the limitations of the fatigue, is a rare gift.

Here are some of the things I have heard over the years about the topic of friendships:

- Some friendships change because of the loss of context – for example, if you leave a job or place of work or can no longer participate in a sports team or fitness class. I have seen successful examples of people maintaining contact by volunteering or becoming a spectator, but, for the majority, it can be a constant and hard reminder of what they are unable to do at the present time.

- Often the larger friendship groups take a back seat for a while, as they are not priority for this season; this can be upsetting at times as people seem to move on with their lives.

- Some friends 'just get it'! They understand something about the fatigue and accept the current situation without demands. Others do not always understand but are open to learn (Tip 6). Friends cannot always guess how you are, so reach out and let them know.

- Flexibility is often needed, as plans change on the day or in the moment. Willingness to adapt is important – for example, watching a football game at home on TV rather than attending the match.

- Many people just like to *be* with others – maybe sitting listening to music, watching TV or a film, doing a jigsaw or having a drink – that is, being relaxed with other people and not having to necessarily make much conversation.

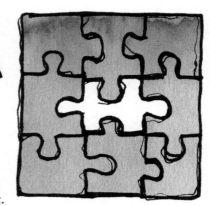

- Try not to rely completely on just one friend.

- Friendships are reciprocal – involving give and take – so be sure to check in with how your friends are and show gratitude for their support.

- Do small low-key sedentary activities together, depending upon your capacity.

- Friends are great companions when you are attempting activities again. They can remind you to take a pacing break or switch your activity because they want you to support your journey to recovery.

> There is a friend who sticks closer than a brother.
> Book of Proverbs[NIV]

TIP 74: APPRECIATE THE GOOD IN OTHERS

We all thrive on authentic appreciation and encouragement. I am not referring to flattery or empty words but truthful appreciation.

> The deepest principle in human nature is the craving to be appreciated.
> William James (1842–1910), founder of American Psychology[2]

I have witnessed countless families break down walls of hostility by the simple act of saying something positive and appreciative to another family member. Thoughtful and simple, yet powerful. One activity that can facilitate this amongst family members, household members or small groups is a simple paper-folding exercise:

- Everyone sits around a table and has an A4 size piece of paper.
- Write your name on the bottom of the paper and pass it to the person on your left.
- Think about something you genuinely appreciate about the person whose name is written on the paper you have.
- Write this at the very top of the paper, then carefully fold the paper over so that no one can see what you have written.
- When you are ready, pass the paper onto the next person and repeat the process.
- You can go round the circle a few times, passing it on again when it comes to your own name.
- When completed, each person can open the paper with their name on it.
- Spend time dwelling on the comments. Any surprises? Any things you had not heard before? Any comments that stand out for you?
- This can also be done with couples.

Many families who have done this exercise in a therapy session continued doing it periodically at home because it can be somewhat life-giving. It also shifts the emphasis from thinking only about the problem and helps to look for the good in others.

- In what ways do you show appreciation?
- In what ways do you receive appreciation?

Every new day is another chance to change your life.
Proverb of unknown origin

TIP 75: DEALING WITH CONFLICTS AND ARGUMENTS AT HOME

We have all been there, done that and got the t-shirt, with regards to having had conflicts and arguments at home. However, I am sure you would agree that home life is sweeter when arguments are absent.

Conflicts can range from being loud and physical to being silent and aloof. Some people may feel better for 'getting it off their chest' and speaking their mind. Sadly though, words that have been spoken briefly in anger usually hurt the deepest and longest and cannot be retracted.

> However conflicts occur, they are always upsetting and exhausting. Emotional energy drains you when your energy is low already. Chronic fatigue affects your levels of tolerance and patience. So how can you communicate what needs to be communicated? How can you deal with difficult issues within the home without it turning into an argument every time? Or communicate without being totally drained?

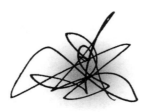

> Every family is different and, as you know already, one size does not fit all (Tip 8). Here are some tools that other families have found useful:

1. If you are in the midst of an argument, try to lower your voice, speak slower, take a physical step back and seek to calm things down.

2. Don't try to resolve the issue in the heat of the moment. Express a desire to talk about the situation when things have calmed down.

3. Do you keep repeating the same kind of arguments over the same kind of things? Is it a similar pattern every time? It is very common in households to do just that, almost

like: 'Oh, here we go again!' Often these arguments accelerate until someone runs out of steam and the issues are usually not resolved. When households recognise this occurring, they have the awareness to decide if they want to continue or not. Some families and couples have given their particular pattern of conflicts an agreed silly name, which any member can shout out in the midst of one. I have heard of some families rolling around in laughter after such an event and other stories of family members still being livid but able to process that at a calmer time. Using this tool prevents spending unnecessary precious energy.

4. Negotiations. Some arguments occur repeatedly over jobs and responsibilities (e.g. taking the dog for a walk, cleaning the bathroom) or over habits (e.g. leaving lights on, spending household money). Talking about these situations, and creating a joint plan that all household members have agreed and contributed to, cuts out the stress.

5. Holding the 'something soft' exercise. This is a simple tool which enables listening skills and can be done when the household is calm. The household member who holds the item can talk without being interrupted. Everyone else must listen. The soft item is passed to the next person who responds to what the first person has said and then says what they want to say and so on. If you have small children, you may want to have a timer. This is a powerful exercise for couples also.

In some households, conflicts and arguments can escalate and lead to abuse. This can be physical, emotional or sexual. Abuse of any kind should not be tolerated or condoned. The above tips are not applicable in those situations. To protect yourself and others in your care you need to get out, seek help and stay safe.

> Better a dry crust with peace and quiet than
> a house full of feasting with strife.
> Book of Proverbs[NIV]

TIP 76: SPOT THE NEGATIVE POINTING FINGER

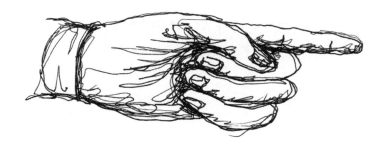

I used to have a laminated pointing finger hand, similar to the illustration above, which I sometimes used in family therapy sessions. The negative pointing finger in relationships can symbolise such things as blame, accusations, criticism, faultfinding, insistence, anger and demands. We all use the negative pointing finger at times, and we have all been on its receiving end.

A lot of upset in relationships can accompany the negative pointing finger too. Often the folks we care for the most get hurt in the process. Words are spoken that cannot be taken back and often other negative pointing fingers, with their effects, appear in response.

Fatigue can cause less tolerance and patience, especially with those you are closest to. Disappointments and frustrations can cause the negative pointing finger to appear more often than we would like. It often takes awareness, energy and humility to deal with them and heal the dynamics. Sadly, negative pointing fingers are not only in our relationships but in almost every sphere of society. You only have to listen to the news, or some gossip on social media, to become more aware of their presence.

Negative pointing fingers can be exhausting.

- Observe the hand in the illustration. Look at the other three fingers – where are they pointing? They are pointing back to the person whose hand it is.

- Take note of pointing fingers in the coming days and weeks. I have worked with people who kept a picture of a pointing finger in their homes; that constant awareness not only saved their energy but also made their homes more peaceful.

Don't jump to conclusions.
Proverb of unknown origin

TIP 77: SUPPORT GROUPS

We all need support in life and dealing with chronic fatigue can be a lonely journey. What I have discovered over the years is that support is a very individual thing – what works for one person may not work for another, but when it works well it is a beautiful thing.

I used to work with many young people, adults and families affected by chronic fatigue who often suffered alone. Some used to comment about how comforting it was to see other people in the waiting room, just to realise that they were not alone. That it was not only them going through this nightmare.

Some people I worked with were part of support groups or Facebook groups and found the support invaluable. Others did not have the energy to initiate social contact wider than their immediate family. Some decided it was not for them and processed their difficulties privately. Others tried a support group and found listening to other people's difficulties more draining than helpful.

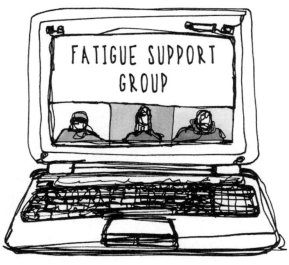

Whilst facilitating group sessions at work, I found that some participants exchanged contact details in the hope of support. Some of those connections provided that support and friendship. Others realised that, despite sharing a diagnosis, their attitude to recovery was completely different and at times the contact became discouraging rather than encouraging.

- Support groups can be wonderful resources to obtain useful information and advice.

- They can point you in a certain direction.
- Some groups have a particular emphasis; be cautious of groups that focus mostly on symptoms and difficulties.
- Voices grouped can often be more powerful than a lone voice if you are seeking reform.
- You can get a flavour of a group by looking at the webpage or online chat. Does it sound like it could help or hinder you in your recovery journey?
- Consider what you would like to discover and learn from others.
- Consider what lessons you have learnt and what you have to share.
- Be careful what you post on social media.

He who suffers much will know much.
Greek proverb

TIP 78: MEDICAL PROFESSIONALS

For this recovery journey, you will need input from medical professionals, such as doctors, nurses and/or therapists. If you have been given a diagnosis of long COVID or CFS/ME, you will already have had blood tests to eliminate other possible causes of your symptoms and potential diagnoses. With long COVID you may also have respiratory or neurological symptoms for which you are under a different specialty consultant, who is monitoring your symptoms. You may also have therapy appointments to facilitate rehabilitation, recovery and management of the symptoms.

Always remember that it is your body. You are, in fact, the expert on your body, but you need professional help at this point. Medical professionals are providing you with a service and offering you their expertise and insights to facilitate your recovery.

> Appointments can be stressful and exhausting. It is your precious time, so do prepare for them to get the most out of the time. I used often to ask people, 'What are you hoping for during this time?'

- Prepare for your appointments.

- Write down things you want to communicate as the health professionals cannot guess; you have to tell them.

- Write down any questions you have.

- If advice is given, take notes or ask to have it written down.

- If an appointment is going to be over 30 minutes, ask for a short pacing break of a few minutes. You might want to bring a drink and/or snack.

- If you do not understand something, do ask.

- If you need support or a second pair of ears, ask if someone can accompany you.

- Most importantly, try to apply the advice you discussed and agreed upon and then give feedback at your next appointment.

A trustworthy envoy brings healing.
Book of Proverbs[NIV]

FOOD FOR THOUGHT

Brené Brown[30] in her book *The Gifts of Imperfection*, discusses the topic of connection. She states:

> I define connection as the energy that exists between people when they feel seen, heard, and valued; when they can give and receive without judgment; and when they derive sustenance and strength from the relationship.*

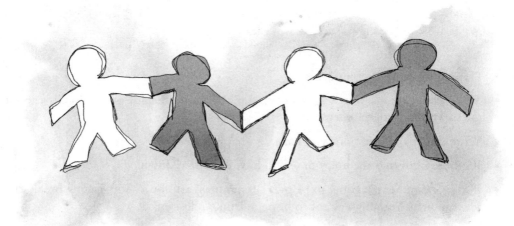

---

*With kind thanks to Brené Brown and her publishers for these words.

PAUSE: WRITE A LETTER

Most of our communication with other people is instant – texts, phone calls, Whatsapp, Facebook messenger, emails. We receive them on our phones wherever we are. This instant correspondence often presumes an immediate response, which can be demanding and difficult for people affected by chronic fatigue. What about the good old handwritten letter or card?

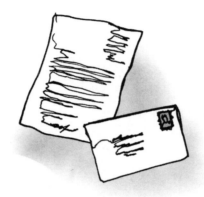

Physical cards and letters, as opposed to electronic ones, can be handled, treasured and reread. They can be short or long, funny or serious, shallow and light or deep and meaningful. They can be written over a few days or all at once. They can be posted, hand-delivered or left for members of your household where they can be found. Often you can express encouraging, thoughtful words more easily on paper than in person. Letters are useful ways to connect with others and have your voice heard, especially when social energy is low.

However a letter is written, the person who receives it knows that someone has thought about them and that, in itself, communicates a lot.

- Keep letters short and sweet.
- Connect with people who come to mind, even members of your own household.
- Encourage and build people up with your words.
- Let them know you are thinking of them.
- Delegate posting the letter if that is too much for you.

MIND, BODY AND SOUL: COMMUNITY AND RELATIONSHIPS

Mind: What were your thoughts as you read this chapter on Community and relationships?

Other parts of the chapter you can let go of for now.

Body: What actions will you start putting into practice?

Soul: You may want to seek soul help with these changes. As explained in the book's Introduction, this section is from my perspective as a Christian, inviting God's help in the recovery process. You may have your own way of seeking soul help, so please do what you feel comfortable with.

Dear God, I ask you for help with community
and relationships and my recovery journey.
'Love is patient, love is kind. It does not boast, it is not proud.
'It does not dishonor others, it is not self-seeking,
it is not easily angered, it keeps no record of wrongs …
'It always protects, always trusts, always hopes,
always perseveres.
'Love never fails.'[NIV]
Thank you God.
Amen — may it be so.
Based upon 1 Corinthians 13[31]

CHAPTER 9

MINDSET — MOOD

Your mood influences so much of your life. If you are feeling happy, you will experience increased motivation and energy. If you are experiencing sadness, and feel somewhat blue, your motivation and energy are automatically depleted. Also vice versa – if your motivation and energy are depleted then you are more likely to feel low and down in mood.

> This illustrates the downward spiral that low mood can follow. This is why it is paramount that you look after your mood, as much as you can.

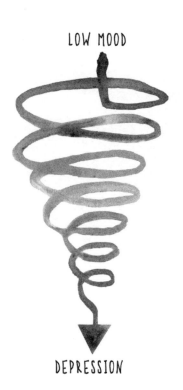

LOW MOOD

DEPRESSION

It can be difficult at times to distinguish between a low mood, depression and chronic fatigue. I have seen patients who have had to convince their local doctor that they were not depressed, but rather fatigued, prior to getting a referral to chronic fatigue services. Many people with CFS/ME do not struggle with depression, but others do. I have also known patients who were referred for a chronic fatigue assessment but required referral to other services since depression was the real issue.

> In fact, there is such an overlap of the symptoms of depression and chronic fatigue that the boundaries often get blurred. Symptoms can be sleep difficulties, low energy, slow movement or speech, neglect of hobbies and interests, intolerant or irritable feelings

towards others, various aches and pains, as well as difficulty in making decisions. Can you recognise the overlap?

Obviously, there are additional symptoms in depression, such as continuous low mood, sadness, tearfulness and, sometimes, suicidal thoughts. Depression fatigue does tend to have a different pattern to chronic fatigue and requires a different emphasis of treatment, hence the importance of knowing which is which.

We all experience low moods from time to time. It is normal that certain life events, such as bereavement, relational breakdowns and conflicts, transitions and adjustments, can cause upset and mood changes. Whether you are currently experiencing a low mood or not, the tips in this chapter cover topics that will enable you to stay mindfully aware of your mood and look after your wellbeing.

TIP 79: TEARS AND SADNESS

There can be many reasons why we cry and many differing responses to our tears. Tears can represent happiness and joy as well as sadness and sorrow. For some people, crying is an unusual occurrence and they have cried only a handful of times in their life. For others, small things, such as a kind word, a gesture, music, a memory or a thought, can readily trigger and cause emotional tears to flow.

> Our body's ability to either hold back the tears or let them flow can often be affected by our mood, hormones, fatigue levels, illnesses and our general sense of wellbeing. Sometimes having a 'good cry' can release tensions and pent-up emotions, followed by a sense of relief and calmness. Emotional tears contain different levels of certain stress hormones compared with other tears. Some researchers have hypothesised that the release of these stress hormones within emotional tears regulates the body and returns balance.[32] There is a time to cry and there is a time to stop crying.

We have all grown up with different narratives around crying. These often shape how comfortable, or not, we are around our own and others' tears and sadness. Also, whether we tend to cry in private or can share our tears with others.

There may be seasons and events in our lives where emotions are raw, and sadness is more present. We may wonder, during those seasons, if the pain and sadness are constantly going to be that extreme, but time can often be a great healer. Life goes on and adjustments occur.

The tears can represent the sadness that perhaps is almost impossible to express in words or process logically in our minds. Often, the last thing we want to be asked is, 'Why are you crying?' Usually, we need empathy, comfort and support expressed in various ways, as well as tissues.

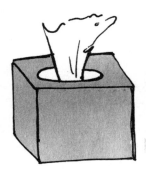

> Sometimes, seasons of crying can go on perhaps too long and get in the way of everyday functioning. Often this can be an indication of needing additional therapeutic help to process the sadness, feel what we feel, increase awareness, accept what is out of our control and take steps to enrich our lives. Be kind to yourself: acknowledge your thoughts and feelings rather than criticising or fighting them.

- Consider, if the tears could speak, what might they say?
- Maybe you could try sharing some of the sadness with someone close?

Tears are, at times, as eloquent as words.
Latin proverb

TIP 80: CONSIDER THE STRESS AND VULNERABILITY BUCKET

The stress and vulnerability bucket[33] can be a helpful concept to consider. Sometimes, sorrows, stress and discouragement can build up in our lives to overflowing, often without our even realising it. The first sign might be a disproportionate reaction to a small trigger, or increasing irritability and tearfulness. It can, at times, feel too much for us to carry on our own.

- Stop and consider what sorrows, stress or discouragements are currently filling your stress and vulnerability bucket. You may want to list them.

- The bucket, representing you, has strength, capability and resilience, but a limited capacity. How are the sorrows, stress and discouragements affecting the bucket at this present moment?

- Do some of the sorrows, stress and discouragements need to be diverted, dealt with or prevented from filling up the bucket in this season? How will you start doing that?

Let us turn our attention to the taps at the bottom of the bucket. The taps, when freely flowing and unblocked, allow the sorrows, stress and discouragements to drain away, decrease or shift. They do not ignore them but do a good job of taking them seriously and not allowing them to be overwhelming or all-consuming.

Taps represent the activities in our lives that help bring balance and they release some of the burdens of the stress and sadness. Everybody's taps are personal and could be such things as talking to others, spending time in nature, maintaining healthy eating, relaxation, family time, hobbies, going for a short walk, or something else. Some of us may have unhealthy taps, such as comfort eating, excessive alcohol or substance misuse or binge-watching TV.

- Stop and consider what your healthy taps are. You may want to list and appreciate each of them.

- Are you able to identify any unhealthy taps and limit their use?

- Are there any healthy taps that perhaps need unblocking and being used more during this season? How will you start doing that?

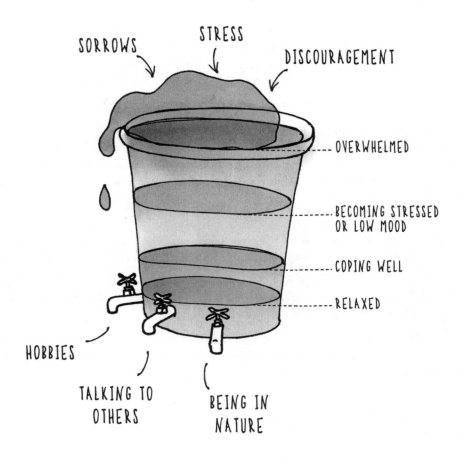

Using this analogy can help make sense of the overwhelming feelings. It can put labels on some thoughts and feelings and also highlight the taps which need to be unblocked and turned on to assist your mood.

> Little by little you fill the sink and
> drop-by-drop you fill the barrel.
> Catalan proverb

TIP 81: LONELINESS AND LOSS

Chronic fatigue can be an extremely lonely affair. At times, it can leave you feeling misunderstood and very alone. Even amid busy households or working and social environments, you can still experience loneliness and isolation. There is something about the importance of being listened to, understood and taken seriously that can cut through this.

Many of my previous patients would often comment about their experience of sitting in the waiting room for the first time. Even though they did not engage in conversation with anyone, they found it surprisingly reassuring to see someone else who was suffering in a similar way and know that they were not alone in their suffering or their journey of recovery.

Anyone who has experienced bereavement knows what loss feels like. The loss of a loved one can be one of the most painful experiences to bear. There are all sorts of losses and adjustments in life, but these include many associated with chronic illness. We tend not to acknowledge or recognise the multiple losses associated with chronic illness. Recognising this and allowing space to process these losses can be an important part of coping with and adapting to the illness. Some are temporary losses and some may be permanent – but each one is personal to you. How you personally cope and adjust to loss may be completely different to how other people do so and that is truly okay.

People's resilience and ability to recreate, adjust and bounce back, with time and healing, never cease to amaze me.

Isolation is a common danger when you experience these thoughts and feelings. In some ways, it may feel like the right thing to do to protect you from any further upset or uncomfortable feelings. In Tip 3: Note your general attitude to illness (page 10), we considered doing things that can feel counterintuitive or the opposite to your natural response, and this can feel wrong and awkward at times. This is one of those situations.

- Take steps towards people – even just to be in the company of others.
- Avoid isolation.
- Talk to others.

- Grieve for some of your losses.
- Be kind to yourself.
- Practise extreme self-care.

Friendship doubles our joy and divides our grief.
Swedish proverb

TIP 82: GUILT

Natural, or genuine, guilt is experienced when a person has done something wrong, such as committing a crime or offending another person, for which they can feel remorseful. Usually, a penalty of time or money is paid for a crime, or humility and asking forgiveness for a relational offence. Despite natural guilt feeling uncomfortable or worse, it usually has a clear cause and effect, with an offence and a penalty.

> Guilty feelings connected to chronic illness are often common-place but not straightforward. This guilt is completely different from natural guilt. I often refer to this kind of guilt as 'false guilt', but you may want to call it something else. The feelings are very real and not false at all but, unlike natural guilt, you have done nothing wrong and yet you still pay a heavy price.

False guilt can plague you for a long time. It is often hard to see where it starts and if there is an end to it. Often, people are unaware that they are carrying this continual load, almost like a bag of heavy stones. I have seen it present in many different ways over the years. At times, it can sound somewhat noble and right and considerate of others, but living under the false burden of guilt is a heavy and exhausting burden to carry.

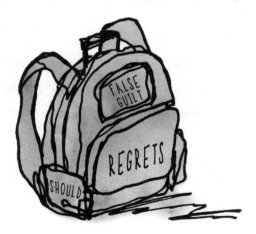

It often includes regrets. Regrets cause us to dwell on things in the past that we *should* or *could* have done. We can certainly learn from the past, but time spent in regret only serves to lower our mood and drain our energy.

Chronic fatigue can bring along all sorts of false guilt, such as:

- Not being well enough.
- Not having enough energy.
- Putting extra burdens on others.
- Needing to cancel plans.
- Being unable to complete certain tasks.
- Taking sick leave from work.
- Letting people down.
- Being known as unreliable.
- Being unable to attend to others' needs as we feel we should.
- Not being the person we were.
- Taking too long to recover.

The list could go on. Emotional energy spent on false guilt and regrets only serves to lower your mood.

- Try to recognise what false guilt you may be carrying.
- Take a moment to notice how this affects you. Possible tension? Sighing? Over-thinking? Does it further lower your mood? Would you judge other people as harshly if they were in your shoes?
- Try to notice without passing judgement or condemning yourself.
- What would you say to a friend who was experiencing similar false guilt?
- This increased awareness may allow you to lay some of the burden down.

Stone is heavy and sand a burden.
Book of Proverbs NIV

TIP 83: CONSIDER PERFECTIONIST TENDENCIES

Perfectionism is an attitude that causes us to keep trying harder. To be perfect, or perform a task perfectly, is impossible and yet we still try. With perfectionism, often the way we feel about ourself – our self-esteem – can be based on our achievements: 'I am good, because I did a good job'.

> Frequently, the standards we set ourselves are too high and unachievable. These unrealistic expectations tend to cause self-blame and criticism that only lead to yet more effort and striving. The striving can be seen as going the extra mile, denying ourselves and our needs. Perfectionist tendencies can also cause procrastination; putting off tasks or never completing them because of the thinking: 'If I complete the project, it may not be good enough'.

Perfectionist tendencies are exhausting

When chronic fatigue comes along and interrupts your life, the energy to maintain those high standards or levels of striving is no longer present. You are unable to achieve what you could perform prior to becoming ill. Your usual standards cannot be met. This in turn knocks your self-esteem and sense of worth. This everyday reality and awareness can be painful, upsetting and frustrating.

People I have worked with over the years who have allowed themselves to feel whatever they feel, even pain or negativity, rather than fighting these negative feelings, apologising for them or feeling guilty for having them, have, with time, done well. Increased awareness of perfectionism and a willingness to embrace more flexibility can often lead to greater levels of freedom from perfectionism.

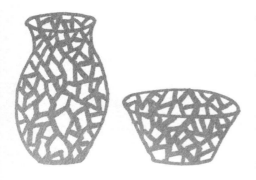

Japanese Kintsugi pottery[34] has often been used as a metaphor for celebrating our uniqueness and embracing our personal imperfections and the many changes that occur throughout our life. The pottery is an ancient art form of repairing broken pottery pieces and transforming them into beautiful showcase pieces. Instead of trying to hide the scars, blemishes and cracks, Kintsugi (translated as 'golden repair') uses gold metal for the repair work. This highlights the cracks, which then become the focus of each piece of pottery.

The pottery is more beautiful and unique than it was prior to being broken and the breakage is part of the object's history.

- Consider this topic of perfectionism: what resonates with you? What feelings or emotions do you notice? Just sit with them for a moment.
- Is there any area of your life where you are setting your standards too high? What could be *just good enough* for this season?
- As you become aware of your self-critic's voice, practise capturing your thoughts (Tip 62).
- Practising thankfulness for small things (Pause: Gratitude: Chapter 9, page 224) and celebrating every small achievements (Tip 35) can help you not only to notice the small things but also to combat the self-critical narrative of not being good enough

> A diamond with a flaw is
> better than a pebble that is perfect.
> Chinese proverb

TIP 84: MEDICATION

Medication for depression has increased significantly over the last few years. There are estimated to be as many as one in seven adults in England currently on prescription antidepressants.[35] I have seen medication give people, affected by depression a helping hand, to lift them somewhat and enable them to see and think a little more clearly.

However, it is not the total answer. I have also seen people put all their hope in medication at the expense of making any healthy lifestyle changes, only to be left in the same situation months later. Medication should always be prescribed and monitored by a doctor and considered as just one component of how to get better.

In the UK, new NICE guidelines for identifying and treating depression in adults[36] are being compiled, at the time of writing. Rather than antidepressants being prescribed straightaway, they are proposing a menu of treatment options, such as talking therapy and gentle exercise, to be discussed with patients first, and medication to be offered only at a later stage.

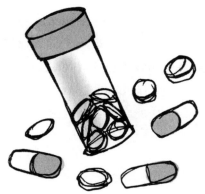

Even in laughter, the heart may ache.
A cheerful heart is a good medicine.
Book of Proverbs[NIV]

TIP 85: WHEN TO GET HELP

> If you recognise that you may need some additional help with your mood, book an appointment with your local doctor. Do it sooner, rather than later, as treatment options such as medication and talking therapies take a while to organise and have an effect. As the downward spiral illustration (at the start of the chapter) shows, if left to continue, a low mood can lead to depression.

Some people try to deal with their confusing emotions and numb feelings on their own and develop DSH (deliberate self harm) as a coping strategy. This can often lead to further isolation and low mood. It is important to seek professional therapy, which can give you the time and space to process your thoughts, feelings and ability to develop healthy alternative coping strategies.

Often people who develop DSH, as an unhealthy coping strategy, really want to feel something and to be alive. Sadly though, depression can also lead other people to suicidal thoughts and attempts to end their life. If this is you, please consider this as an emergency and take the courageous step of telling someone immediately and getting the help and support you currently need.

> You cannot prevent the birds of sadness from passing over your head, but you can prevent them from nesting in your hair.
> Swedish proverb

TIP 86: PRACTISE EXTREME SELF-CARE

We are all familiar with the phrase 'extreme sports' to describe spectacular activities that involve high levels of adrenaline and risk. These sports require total dedication, repetitive practice and complete commitment because the person's life literally depends upon mastering the necessary skills.

In the same way, we can consider extreme self-care. Our wellbeing, mood and recovery depend upon it. I have seen this time and time again. People who prioritise their health and recovery (Tip 34), no matter what the cost, tend to do better than those who do not.

Some people are put off by the phrase self-care as it may sound like self-indulgence or crass selfishness. Just to address that false notion, it is all about balance and being able to steward and look after your health and body for recovery and the long term. For this season of recovery, and especially if you are experiencing a low mood, it is essential and one of the best medicines. It is also a generous gesture towards those you love and care about, as they will undoubtedly be worried about you.

So, what is extreme self-care? What does it look like?

I have recently had the tremendous joy of becoming a grandparent for the first time. As I look at this beautiful, vulnerable little baby and see all the multiple ways his parents not only care for his immediate needs (to sleep, be fed and be cleaned) but also *soothe him* (by rocking, cuddling, stroking and singing) and *enjoy* him (by laughing, playing and talking). I see how vital soothing and enjoying him are for his wellbeing and development.

> Extreme self-care does not only include meeting our basic needs but also involves *soothing activities* and *enjoyable activities*. These often get left out with any chronic illness as all one's energy is spent on trying to get through the day. These activities do not need to take up much time; in fact, over the years the activities I have heard about are usually very short but very sweet to the person concerned.

Soothing activities often involve the senses: the fragrant hand cream, the body scrub in the bath, the after-shave aroma, the hot water bottle, the glow of a candle, the talking book, the weighted blanket, the rocking chair, the same old song that makes you smile, the photographs that evoke happy thoughts, the healthy snack that brings back good memories. All these will be personal to each of us. Activating our senses, in this gentle, tender way, can calm us down, cheer us up and literally soothe us. Some people keep a box of soothing activities and perhaps explore their box for 5-10 minutes each day.

The English National Opera, in conjunction with healthcare teams, has developed a breathing and wellbeing programme for post COVID patients called ENO Breathe.[37] It focuses on breathing retraining through singing. Interestingly, they use lullabies specifically because they calm and soothe us. Breathing exercises also stimulate the vagus nerve.[25] (See 'Pause: Breathe from your diaphram' on page 178).

Enjoyable activities need only to be for 5-10 minutes each day to have an effect. Choosing to do them is giving us permission to enjoy and do something for ourselves. It may be knitting, playing a musical instrument, doing a few pieces of a jigsaw, applying makeup, drawing, playing chess, watching a funny animal clip from YouTube, carpentry – whatever works for you.

- Spend some time considering what soothing and enjoyable activities you could start putting into practice for 5-10 minutes each day.

- Make a list of your Happy Dos – your little Yeses.

- Start to put together your own box and try some soothing activities.

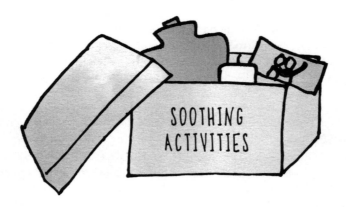

One joy can drive away a hundred sorrows.
Japanese proverb

FOOD FOR THOUGHT

The 'mind bully' is a useful metaphor[38] frequently used in therapy. It represents a particular problem you are struggling with.

You are standing on one side of a large pit and the mind bully, who is big and strong, is on the opposite side. You are both holding one end of a rope, pulling back and forth over the pit. The mind bully is constantly attempting to pull you into the pit.

As with any bully, the mind bully can only harm you when you choose to engage with it and believe the negative things it says. Whenever you pull on the rope, you are in fact feeding the mind bully by listening, paying attention and at times believing it.

The less you feed the mind bully, the smaller and more insignificant it will become. I wonder what would happen if you managed to drop the rope instead of pulling it? You could just put the rope down and turn away.

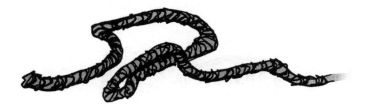

The mind bully may still be there, shouting its insults and hurtful remarks. You can still acknowledge and notice it, but by dropping the rope you are shifting your attention away from it and no longer believing what it says. You are not letting it bully you anymore.

PAUSE: GRATITUDE

Stopping to be thankful is also part of reflecting (Tip 14).

Reflecting is a useful and necessary exercise to help pace your activities. It enables you to consider what works, what does not and what needs to change.

Each evening, stop and look back on your day for a short while:

- What went well?

- What did you do well?

- What or who are you grateful for?

Some people choose to keep a gratitude diary, noting specific things from their day. This helps focus on solutions and positives, rather than on problems.

Ending your day with reflection and thankfulness, no matter how difficult it may have been, positions you in a place of gratitude, ready for what the next day might hold.

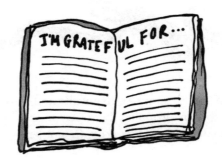

MIND, BODY AND SOUL: MINDSET – MOOD

Mind: What were your thoughts as you read this chapter on Mindset: Mood?

You can let go of other parts of the chapter for now.

Body: What actions will you start putting into practice?

Soul: You may like to seek soul help with these changes. As explained in the book's Introduction, this section is from my perspective as a Christian, inviting God's help in the recovery process. You may have your own way of seeking soul help, so please do what you feel comfortable with.

Dear God, I ask you for help with my mood
and my recovery journey.
Grant me the serenity to accept the things
I cannot change, courage to change the things I can,
and wisdom to know the difference.
Thank you, God.
Amen — may it be so.
The Serenity Prayer[39]

CHAPTER 10

ADDITIONAL HELP

As you continue on your recovery journey, you will experience the benefits of putting the principles of pacing into practice and they will become more natural and automatic.

There are some issues along the way that may require additional help, focus and attention. When these are dealt with, the journey of recovery continues, but when not, these issues or symptoms can become a large hurdle to overcome. This can seem so unfair given all that you have achieved so far.

When considering additional help, a useful analogy is that of professional tennis players in a match at Wimbledon. They know the game well, just as you know pacing well by now, but they still require additional help:

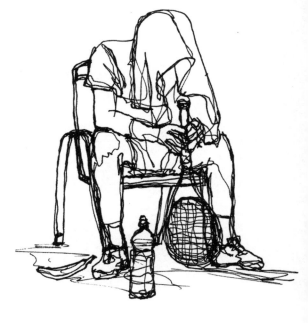

- they consume energy-giving snacks and drinks during the breaks.

- players may sit with a towel over their head, giving themselves a short break on their own.

- they may require treatments from specialist physiotherapists.

- some players wear joint braces, or strapping, to provide additional support and stability.

Occasionally, during a match, they need additional specific help in order to complete the tournament; in a similar way, you may need additional specific help to continue your recovery journey.

The additional help discussed in this chapter covers tips that others have found useful for dealing with certain annoying symptoms and certain life situations. Some will be applicable to your particular circumstances and others may not be.

TIP 87: BRAIN FOG

Cognitive dysfunction, or 'brain fog' as it is more commonly known, is a very common symptom. It is mental fatigue and most sufferers, to some degree, experience it. For some, it is their most disabling symptom.

> If you have experienced brain fog, you know exactly what I am describing. If you have not, it is extremely difficult to describe adequately in words. It can be frightening, and overwhelming, to find that at any given moment you are not able to think straight, function cognitively or produce the words that you know are there.
>
> **Be assured that you are not going mad.**
>
> Brain fog is a fluctuating symptom and worsens with tiredness. It mirrors the fatigue pattern of 'good and bad days'. The good news is that, unlike dementia, brain fog is not a progressive illness. It is a symptom of long COVID fatigue, and CFS/ME. Managing this fatigue, as per all the tips in this book, is the most effective way to influence brain fog.

Sustained mental activity is necessary for most everyday tasks. Brain fog, which is a form of cognitive dysfunction, impacts everything we do. It affects concentration, attention, information processing, planning, organising, sequencing, problem solving, decision making, memory and word-finding abilities. Struggling to find the correct word in conversation is common, as is mixing up commonly used words or using another word which starts with the same letter – for example, *'I was born in Wimbledon'* rather than *'I was born in Windermere'*. Or reordering a sentence construction – for example, *'I need to take the microwave out of the food'* rather than *'I need to take the food out of the microwave'*. It is particularly frustrating and embarrassing because we know that it is incorrect.

Practical tips:

- Reassure yourself that you are not going mad; stress and anxiety only make brain fog worse.
- Sleep, a healthy diet and pacing are crucial to managing brain fog.
- Do your cognitive tasks in very small chunks, even though it may interrupt

your flow and be difficult to re-focus again.

- Practise switching between small chunks of cognitive and physical activity.

- Your physical energy may have improved a lot more than your cognitive energy, so aim to apply all the principles of Chapters 5 and 6 to your cognitive energy.

- Be organised and make sure you put things where they can be easily found.

- Clear clutter so that you are not distracted.

- Drink plenty of water (Tip 47).

- Use visual cues: highlighters, coloured notes, lists, reminders.

- Try not to avoid social situations, but keep them short and simple.

- Discover what is mentally relaxing for you: perhaps listening to instrumental or classical music, or doing Pilates rather than watching TV?

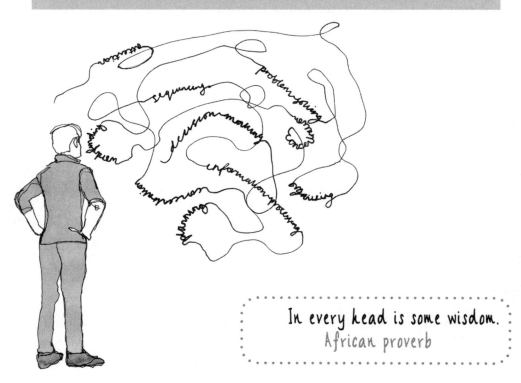

In every head is some wisdom.
African proverb

TIP 88: MANAGE THE PAIN

Persistent pain can scream so loudly that, at times, it is impossible to give your attention to anything else. When I worked in a Pain Management service, we used the metaphor of pain being like a volume switch on the loudest setting. The important thing was learning how to turn it down.

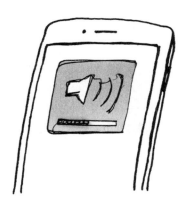

Pain is all too real. Often the body heals but the brain continues to produce pain responses from an injury. This means it is possible to manage the pain without causing further damage. These are examples of how people have turned their pain volume switch down:

- Concentrate on fatigue recovery: pain gets worse when the fatigue is worse (Tip 13).

- Pacing and activity management: the treatment for persistent pain is almost identical to treatment for chronic fatigue. All the tips in this book relating to fatigue also can be applied to pain.

- Active acceptance (Tips 33, 94).

- Get to know the pain and its strategies:

  - What helps?
  - Warmth, gentle movement?

  - What hinders?
  - Overdoing, underdoing, being tired?

- Pain often causes you to stop, so keep moving and stretching, little and often, and avoid deconditioning.

- Learn to relax.

- Ask a doctor to assess the pain, as medication can be an option but only when used in conjunction with self-management.

- Look after your whole body: focus on your sleep, diet and physical and mental health.

It is more painful to do nothing than something.
German proverb

TIP 89: PoTS

Postural orthostatic tachycardia syndrome is a collection of symptoms that some people with chronic fatigue also experience. My observation has been that it often, but not exclusively, affects tall, thin females.

The main symptoms of PoTS are experienced when sitting up from lying flat or standing up from sitting. The change in posture increases the heart rate, which causes dizziness or fainting, and possibly heart palpitations, difficulty with temperature regulation, headaches and shortness of breath. For the person affected it can be debilitating. It can undermine your confidence, and your family's, in your mobility. What if I fall? Am I safe to go down the stairs or go outside?

> If you think you may be struggling with PoTS, ask for an assessment from your medical doctor. I have noticed that understanding what it is and how it can be managed can really help. Advice often includes:

- Drink plenty of water/fluids.

- Always sit up slowly from lying down, then stay seated for a while before gradually standing up.

- Avoid caffeine, alcohol and nicotine.

- If you do not consume much salt in your diet, include more salt but take advice from your doctor.

- If dizzy, lie down for a short period, with your feet elevated.

- If dizzy, move and clench your hands and feet to encourage circulation.

- Maintain a low temperature in the bedroom, perhaps with an electric fan.

> **Headaches need soup.**
> Sicilian proverb

TIP 90: SETBACKS

Setbacks, or relapses, are all par for the course in this recovery journey, due to the fluctuating nature of chronic fatigue. Setbacks are when you feel ill and your symptoms are aggravated. The main advice seasoned recoverers would give you, would be:

- Don't panic and stick to a routine.

The quickest way to turn a setback around is to stick with your fatigue management strategies.

Sometimes it is obvious why a setback has occurred. Perhaps you overdid it for a few days or caught a virus? At other times, there is no clear reason, which can be disconcerting, but the advice would still be the same.

Some people may become discouraged and feel like they are right back at the start, but they soon realise that time and experience have given them the expertise they need. They then must choose either to submit to the fatigue or to turn things around, by downgrading everything (Tip 58), taking additional preventative rests (Tip 51), continuing with pacing and, most importantly, continuing with balanced and realistic routines.

- Don't panic, and try to stay positive.
- Downgrade everything for a short while.
- Go back to basics and follow the tips which helped you the most at the start of your journey.
- Stay in a healthy routine, especially with regard to sleep.

Usually, setbacks can be turned around quickly. With time and practice, you will notice that both the duration of the setbacks, and their frequency, will decrease.

> Salvage something from every setback.
> English proverb

TIP 91: HAVE A GRADED RETURN TO WORK

Many people return to work before they are fully better. This is understandable, given the pressure of job responsibilities, finances and the desire for normality. However, returning to work too soon can cause a relapse, post-exertion malaise and enforced sick leave.

A recent large international research study*with participants affected by long COVID captured some of the participants' comments regarding the severe impact the illness had on their work:

'I worked at some point for a few weeks, in June, but had to stop (couldn't handle a conversation on the phone without brain fog/feeling dizzy/heavy breath trouble because of talking) after a few minutes.'

'Haven't been able to work for ... months due to brain fog. Was supposed to go back last week on reduced hours. I resigned instead. I have worked there as Director of ... for just over ... years.'

'Still on medical leave. Unpaid and denied short term disability.'

'I went from being a workaholic to no work at all. This is the extreme opposite of who I am. I do not know the person I have become.'

'I went back to work too soon and wish I hadn't. I finally had to take a five-week break in July/August with the support of my employer. This helped a lot. I have now been back at work for five weeks and my symptoms have got worse to a degree.'

'I had to take two weeks off, had to work from home for four, but had to return for two weeks with fever as my employer would not give me more time.'

'I asked to reduce hours or work more from home, which was denied.'

'I've been working from home. Haven't officially reduced my hours, but my boss has been flexible and encouraged me to rest when needed.'

---

*With kind thanks to the authors of this paper for giving open access to their work.

'While I've been able to keep my job while working from home, I must admit that if it were not so, I would most definitely NOT be able to work at all. I can barely leave my bedroom on most days.'

'I have needed more flexible hours (working remotely) post-COVID. That way, I can rest as needed throughout the day. If I had to return to in-person work at this point, it would be severely reduced hours if at all.'

As you can see, returning to work can be a difficult process. Everyone is completely different, in terms of severity of illness, recovery, job demands and flexibility. Fatigue recovery usually takes a long time but the longer you are off work, the harder a return may be.

Some points to consider include:

- Keep your line manager at work updated on your situation. Do not expect them to be fully informed of your condition; you may need to signpost them to some information on fatigue.

- Talk to your doctor/health worker. Seek their opinion about returning to work and your current level of capacity.

- Different countries have different work fitness schemes or policies. Try to access occupational health advice regarding any changes that an occupational therapist would recommend for both yourself and your workplace.

- Consider all the small details of your job. What adaptations (Tip 54) in terms of time (Tip 43), environment (Tip 44) and activity (Tip 45) could make your job manageable? Consider your commute to and from work. Write your ideal list – for example, more breaks, a quieter working environment, flexible working hours, home working.

- If you have return to work meetings, consider having somebody accompany you – friend, family member or union official.

- A graded return to work in the UK is normally over a six-week period. Make sure that you have made significant progress already before attempting it. In terms of fatigue rehabilitation, six weeks is a short time.

- In the weeks leading up to your return, start to mimic your working day routine, keeping in place the healthy habits you have been developing.

- Once you have started your phased return, initially you will feel tired, so protect yourself from crashing on your days off – evaluate and downgrade if necessary (Tip 58).

From little acorns mighty oaks do grow.
British proverb

TIP 92: EDUCATION

For many children, adolescents and young adults, education is the equivalent to work. Juggling fatigue symptoms with learning, studying and examinations can be extremely challenging. Attending and participating in school, college or university requires physical, social/emotional and cognitive energy. Learning requires concentration, information processing and memory, all of which are affected by fatigue.

Examinations and progression of course programs continue; they do not wait. Absenteeism only compounds the difficulties, and the amount of work to catch up on increases.

As with work (Tip 91), many young people return to fulltime education too soon and often end up experiencing post-exertion malaise and crashing every evening and all weekend. Many young people struggle to attend fulltime education. In my experience, the most successful integrations back to school have involved staying engaged with school and initially being on a partial timetable.

Some useful tips include:

- Promptly consider a partial timetable.

- Have a small amount of work sent home.

- Practise and continue pacing with all academic work (Tip 56).

- If possible, drop some subjects for this season.

- Find a balance between academic activities and social activities.

- Seek a named person/mentor in the educational establishment.

- Apply for any concessions, such as extra time in exam situations or with submission deadlines.

- Ask for access to a quiet room/space.

- When experiencing more energy, plan a graded return and support for re-integrating.

- Keep brain fog in check (Tip 87).

> Learning is a treasure, which
> accompanies its owner everywhere.
> Chinese proverb

TIP 93: INCREASED SENSITIVITIES

A lot of people, but not everyone with chronic fatigue, also suffer from increased sensitivity to certain things. Often the more fatigue you experience, on any given day, the stronger the sensitivity may be. Over time I have seen this presented in different ways, affecting all five senses:

Light sensitivity: Low tolerance for bright lights, especially indoor fluorescent lighting, sunlight, screens, monitors and phones. *Wear sunglasses and baseball-type caps. Change computer screen brightness; switch on blue-light filters on devices. Use soft lighting and lamps indoors.*

Noise sensitivity: Difficulty coping with noise. Background noise is too loud, distracting and intrusive as it not only makes concentration difficult but it is also irritating and provokes headaches. *Wear earmuffs, earplugs and headphones where appropriate, and choose relaxing music and quieter environments.*

Smell sensitivity: Previously pleasant smells or fragrances are now unpleasant. COVID also causes loss of smell and taste for some people. *Access smell or olfactory training, as this may be helpful.*

Taste sensitivity: Loss of taste of certain foods or unpleasant tastes. *Continue to eat a balanced diet. Avoid foods that taste unpleasant but try them again in a week. Experiment with different temperatures of food. Add stronger-tasting ingredients – sour, sweet, bitter and salty.*

Skin sensitivity: Discomfort with certain clothes and materials on your skin, which is experienced more with persistent pain conditions rather than chronic fatigue. *Seek to gradually desensitise the area by regularly, and gently, touching the skin with different textured materials.*

Temperature regulation: Hot and cold temperature regulation changes. *Wear thin layers that can be easily taken on and off.*

Dietary sensitivities: Different food intolerances, either developed or discovered since chronic fatigue. *Seek dietitian's advice and possibly trial elimination diets.*

Alcohol sensitivity: Tolerance for alcohol decreases and you only need to drink a small amount to feel slightly drunk. This can be especially difficult when starting to socialise again. *Be aware of this before socialising.*

Hormone sensitivity: Some women report exacerbated fatigue during menstruation. *Plan and anticipate lowered energy/emotional stamina. Downgrade (Tip 58) for that week whilst continuing your daily routine.*

Most of these strategies attempt to avoid stimulation but, as your energy begins to recover, it can help to gradually try and expose yourself to relevant stimuli that you may have been avoiding, and consider their effects on you.

> Peace is costly but it is worth the expense.
> African proverb

TIP 94: TRY MINDFULNESS

Mindfulness is a secular practice that enables you to become more aware of what you experience in the present moment. It helps you to be *fully awake* right now – not in the future or in the past. This includes internal awareness of your body, thoughts, emotions, feelings plus external noises, smells, textures and warmth. It allows you to notice and hold those experiences lightly, with an attitude of care, curiosity and openness, rather than judgement or criticism.

> With long COVID fatigue, or CFS/ME, you may at times feel like running away from all the physical symptoms, thoughts, feelings and emotions, but that could lead to the fatigue having greater control. Slowing down, and increasing your awareness of the present moment, may help you to turn towards unpleasant experiences more gently and compassionately. From this stepped-back position of awareness and kindness, you can have moments of choice, rather than being driven by habitual reactions.

I have worked with many people who have tried mindfulness. Some have tried it and it has not been for them and others have done so with transformative effects on their life. It is not a substitute for pacing and activity management, but it can certainly enrich and add to your outlook, freedom, health and wellbeing.

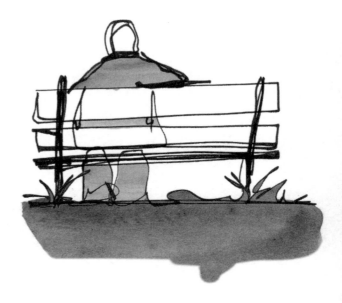

There is so much in the public arena about mindfulness that it is difficult to know where to start, but here are some useful suggestions:

- Try a shorter practice (5-10 minutes) such as the 'Pause: Mindfulness body scan practice for sleep' on page 78.

- Experiment with watching or listening to material by a qualified mindfulness teacher or reputable organisation, such as Mindfulness: Finding peace in a frantic world.

- Listen to some of the audio scripts available online.

- If you wish to pursue it, consider joining a local sitting group, either online or in-person.

- Be playful and experiment with a variety of mindfulness practices (breathing, body scan, sounds, etc) but also know that you do not need to persist with any practice that feels too much. Remember that you are the expert on your body.

> Whoever is patient has great understanding.
> Book of Proverbs [NIV]

TIP 95: CONSIDER VOLUNTEERING

If you are not currently in employment or education, this tip may be worth considering. I have seen many people, who are usually some way down the road to recovery, benefit greatly from volunteering.

People start volunteering for many different reasons. Some are reasonably fit and able, but perhaps unsure of their energy capacity for employment. Some want to make a contribution and to have contact with people. Others use it to gain experience and confidence before seeking employment. The benefits, such as routine, responsibility, self-belief, confidence, team-working, and contribution to a bigger cause, can be rewarding in ways that you have not anticipated.

Volunteering roles vary enormously, but each carries responsibility. The main difference between volunteering and employment is that you are giving your time freely. Before you start in any position, you should consider what you are willing and able to give and what situation would be conducive for your ongoing recovery. For example, I have seen people who have negotiated with charity shops to work only a few hours a day, initially twice a week with breaks, and then gradually build this up to longer days.

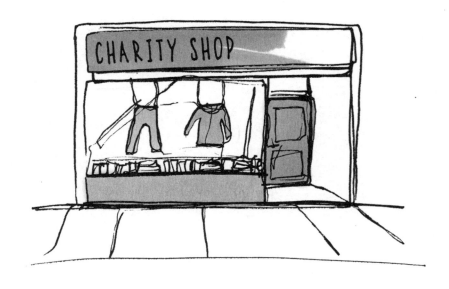

- Before rushing to volunteer, gradually build up your capacity.

- Mimic the volunteer's role at home – for example, perhaps stand for 30 minutes, or combine social and cognitive activity, such as talking and working at a till.

- Consider your limits and how you can apply pacing within this role.

- Choose somewhere close to home and allow time for pacing within your journey.

> One volunteer is better than 10 forced men.
> African proverb

TIP 96: WEBSITES AND BLOGS

Isn't it amazing that we can access almost any information from all over the world, instantly and directly on our phones and computers? There is more information available at our fingertips than in any previous generation.

> The Internet contains the good, the bad and the ugly. In the early stages of recovery, many people I have worked with have spent hours searching the Internet, consulting 'Dr Google' to check their symptoms and seek a cure or a way forward. Even though the Internet is amazing, we can all experience information overload.

This can also be the case for relatives, partners and parents. I have met exhausted relatives who have spent many late nights constantly searching, to little or no avail. Often, it is an act of love and desire to help and bring about the much-needed change. Sometimes this can prove fruitful and useful. Other times, it can be exhausting and anxiety-provoking and sometimes it can actually be counter-productive for recovery.

The positive side of the Internet is the amazing connection it gives to others. Many socially isolated people can participate in online chats and be in contact with many people across the globe, without the need to travel. Through the pandemic, even the technologically challenged have come to rely on this form of communication.

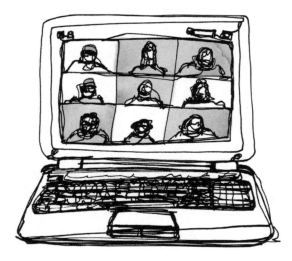

Considerations for searching the Internet include:

- Clarify what you are hoping to find out.

- Do you have a sense of peace and re-assurance, or increased fear and anxiety, after being online?

- Are the blogs, stories and examples you are reading, encouraging and perhaps challenging you to keep on the recovery journey or are they having a negative effect?

- Remember to pace, take breaks and switch activities.

- Avoid late evening online searches or communications.

- Make wise choices about computer use; limit your time and your searches and remember that you are spending your precious energy coins (Tip 39, Tip 46).

- If brain fog (Tip 87) is an ongoing symptom for you, delegate any searches you want to do and ask for a summary.

> Knowledge is a treasure, but practice is the key to it.
> Arab proverb

FOOD FOR THOUGHT

An extensive research study entitled 'Characterizing long COVID in an International Cohort: 7 Months of Symptoms and Their Impact', surveyed 3762 respondents affected by long COVID from 56 countries.*[40] The objective of this study was to characterise the symptom profile of patients with long COVID, along with the impact of the condition on daily life, work and return to baseline health.

The following is a quote from the study about the **impact on work**:

'*Of unrecovered respondents who worked before becoming ill, only 27.3% were working as many hours as they were prior to becoming ill at the time of survey, compared to 49.3% of recovered respondents. Nearly half (45.6%) of unrecovered respondents were working reduced hours at the time of the survey, and 23.3% were not working at the time of the survey as a direct result of their illness. This included being on sick leave, disability leave, being fired, quitting, and being unable to find a job that would accommodate them. The remaining respondents retired, were volunteers, or did not provide enough information to determine their working status. Overall, 45.2% of respondents reported requiring a reduced work schedule compared to pre-illness. 22.3% were not working at the time of survey due to their health conditions.*

At least 45% of working respondents were working remotely at the time of the survey, and it was noted how critical this was to respondents' continued ability to work. Teleworking enabled respondents to take breaks when necessary and saved them the physical exertion of commuting to work. Respondents mentioned asking for other accommodations at work like flextime or moving to a role with lower physical or mental strain. Even with telecommuting, phased returns, and other accommodations, respondents commented on how difficult it was for them to work full or part-time, but described their financial need to do so.

It is important to note that the survey captured only a moment in time. Respondents described taking months of leave before going back to work either full-time or at reduced hours. Further, there were respondents who indicated that they tried to go back to work for several weeks but then relapsed or were unable to complete their work satisfactorily.

---

*With kind thanks to the authors of this paper for giving open access to their work.

PAUSE: LAUGHTER

At some point in our lives, we have all experienced the positive effects of having a good laugh. The laughs I remember most are those with other people. Everyone laughing, almost to the point of crying, and whatever it was that caused the laughter is almost irrelevant.

Times of laughter can be hard to find in the midst of chronic illness. Over the years, I have noticed the beneficial effects of patients having an authentic positive attitude and a sense of humour. With some people, it comes naturally and perhaps is part of the home environment, but with other people, I have seen clear choices and intentionality to choose positivity and humour.

Laughter has many positive effects on your physical body and your mental health. Practise being intentional about positivity and laughter:

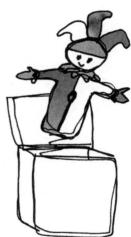

- Smile more.

- Watch a funny film or YouTube clip.

- If energy permits, play a short game.

- Practise being thankful.

- Although hard to do, try replacing self-criticism, towards some of your mistakes, with laughter.

- Bring humour into your conversations by asking questions such as, 'What is the funniest thing that ever happened to you?' or 'What funny joke have you heard recently?'

MIND, BODY AND SOUL: ADDITIONAL HELP

Mind: What were your thoughts as you read this chapter on Additional help?

Other parts of the chapter you can let go of for now.

Body: What actions will you start putting into practice?

Soul: You may like to seek soul help with these changes. As explained in the book's Introduction, this section is from my perspective as a Christian, inviting God's help in the recovery process. You may have your own way of seeking soul help, so please do what you feel comfortable with.

Dear God, I ask you for help with additional
help and my recovery journey.
You say — 'Do not fear, for I am with you ...
'I will strengthen you and help you;
'I will uphold you ...
'I myself will help you.' NIV
Thank you God.
Amen — may it be so.
Based upon Isaiah 41[41]

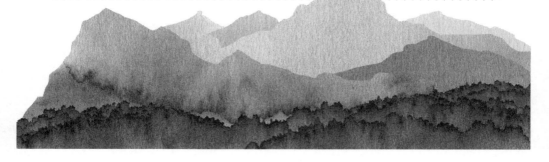

CHAPTER 11

MAINTAINING PROGRESS – YOUR FUTURE

Wherever you currently are on your road to recovery, you have made progress. You may consider your progress to be immense or minuscule. Whatever your self-assessment may be regarding your progress, you are now in a different place to where you were at the start of your journey.

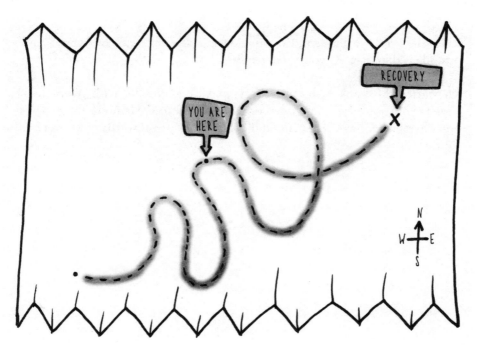

The journey with fatigue, as you know, has many stops and starts, many twists and turns and many ups and downs. You now have more expertise and awareness about the fatigue and its strategies and, more importantly, how it affects you personally.

You are learning the importance of good sleep habits, realistic routines, taking small steps, healthy eating and balancing your energy levels and activities for your physical, and mental, health and wellbeing. Not only are you learning about these skills theoretically but also practically. You have had to come back to them, time and time again, and repeat them in order to experience their benefit. There is no quick fix and most of your efforts will have gone unseen and unknown – but that is what it has taken to get this far.

Many people who have come to the end of their therapy sessions are not 'fully better'; they still have a way to go. The majority have the self-confidence to handle the fatigue and get on with their lives and continue their steady progress. Some may have made major adjustments to their lives, reduced their hours at work, changed jobs and now be living a simpler, more balanced life. Others may have experienced the joy of, and renewed appreciation for, being able to do certain long-forgotten activities again. For many, the continual practice of reflecting, being present in the moment, mindfully aware and making healthy choices will have become a lifestyle. Some people in their recovery may have even wanted to become undiagnosed and not to wear the label of illness anymore, although this is often harder than it sounds.

> Everyone's story is different. Everyone's progress is different. Everyone's attitude is different. As yours will be too.
>
> We started this book with 'Your story' and we will end it with 'Your story'. This is your journey, your recovery and your future. Maintain the progress you have made, however small, and continue to step towards your preferred future.

TIP 97: CONTINUE REFLECTING, PACING AND LOOKING FORWARDS

'I never thought it would work but it really does.' I have heard these words, or similar, more times than I can even begin to recall. They never cease to put a smile on my face.

In all honesty, the concept of pacing is very simple. There is nothing complicated about it. However, amid all the uncertainty, fatigue, pain and horrendous symptoms, I can understand people thinking that it will not work. Thinking that maybe they need a more prescriptive approach or some medicine, or medical intervention.

As much as pacing is an easy concept, it is incredibly difficult to put into practice. I respect each of you for being willing to give it a go. Everyone who has persevered with pacing will reach a point where they realise that it does work. They may experience that it is helping them to deal quickly with a setback or extreme post-exertion malaise. Perhaps they begin to wake up on consecutive days and feel slightly healthier. Maybe their head starts to feel clearer, little by little. Or they manage to attend a social event without crashing afterwards. Overall, they can see the benefits to their energy levels gradually increasing over time, little by little.

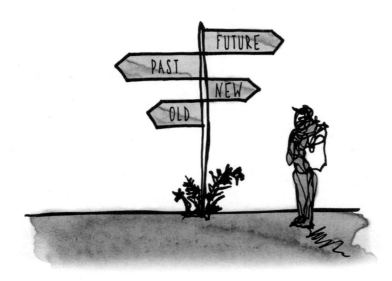

This is what pacing does and this is how pacing works – little by little.

I wonder what your experience is so far? I hope that you have reached the point of recognising that pacing works for you and that you are starting to experience its benefits in your everyday life. If not yet, it will come, little by little.

> Give careful thought to the paths of your feet.
> Book of Proverbs[NIV]

TIP 98: TRY THE WHEEL OF LIFE TOOL

For this season, you need to prioritise your health. Experiencing chronic fatigue comes with a high personal price, which affects all areas of your life. Sadly, there is no getting away from that fact. However, you have been making healthy choices and are rebuilding your life.

The Wheel of Life can be a useful tool to use every few months. It gives a holistic overview of different areas of your life and can enable you to evaluate your priorities for the present season, as well as give guidance for the future.

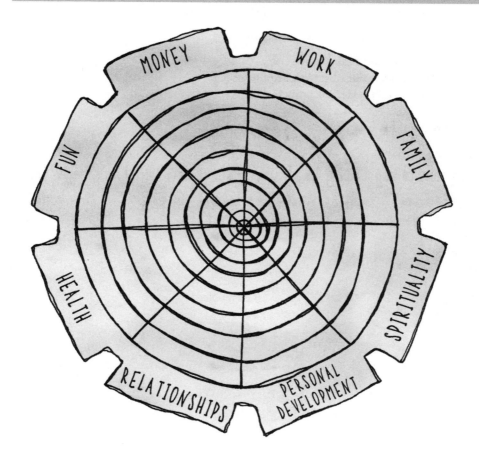

- Consider what each category in the Wheel means to you. Are there any other categories you wish to add or change? For example, 'money' can also mean the opportunities you have or the environment you live in, which depends upon money. 'Spirituality' may imply hope, peace or guidance for you.

- Rank each category in priority order e.g. Health = 1, Family = 2, Work = 3, etc, with '1' being 'most important'.

- Taking one category at a time, mark on the concentric circles between 1-10:

  a. What your present reality is.
  b. Where you would like it to be, realistically.

- When complete, ask yourself:

  a. What do I notice? Are there any surprises?
  b. Do I want to rearrange any of the priorities, or not?

- For each category, now ask yourself:

  a. What would make it better?
  b. What potential obstacles are there?
  c. Are there any action points?

Plan to review this in a few months (see Appendix 4).

> Do something today that your future self will thank you for.
> Proverb of unknown source

TIP 99: HAVE YOUR PROGRESS WITNESSED – TAKE PART IN RESEARCH

There is still so much unknown about COVID-19, long COVID and CFS/ME. In this book, we have focused on the most dominant symptom of long COVID – the chronic fatigue – as this has an impact on everything else.

The tips within these pages have come from over 15 years of experience, witnessing hundreds of people walk this recovery path, one small step at a time. Hopefully, you have benefited from their hard-earned experience.

Despite chronic health conditions costing health services more[42] in the long term, chronic fatigue services have often been overlooked and under-resourced. Over the years, we have had to fight to keep services alive and to justify their existence.

> Due to the global impact of COVID-19 and the millions of lives that have been severely affected by long COVID, there are now, more than ever before, multiple research studies into long COVID and accompanying symptoms such as chronic fatigue. These are seeking to find causes, solutions and ways forward.

In the midst of all the chaos, pain, loss and uncertainty, this provides some hope. By writing this book, my intention is to offer you, the reader, some hope and clear pointers forward regarding the horrendous fatigue.

Similarly, I hope that research will provide solutions soon for so many people struggling with this condition.

- Consider contributing your stories and experience for research purposes.
- Ask your local doctor if there are any research projects you can participate in.
- Realise that your story may help others, so do not underestimate the power of joining with other voices to share your experience.

Shared joy is double joy. Shared sorrow is half sorrow.
Swedish proverb

TIP 100: WHAT TIPS WOULD YOU GIVE?

You have come this far on your recovery journey. Well done! I wonder, as you reflect, which tips have been the most useful for you.

During the final sessions of therapy with a patient, I often asked them the following question:

> • If a friend received a diagnosis of chronic fatigue, what top five tips would you share with them?
>
> This is a useful exercise to do, as listing these personal priority tips usually crystallises what is most useful for you. Obviously, you can have more than five tips. Some people choose to call their personal list a 'First Aid Plan', 'Setback Plan' or 'Relapse Plan'.

Whatever you choose to call it, it is:

- what you have practised and experienced to get you to where you are now.
- what will help you to get back on track if you go too fast or too slowly.
- what will help you gradually recover from any crashes.
- what will continue to enable you to improve.

As I bring this book to a close, I also wonder if you have any other tips of your own that you find useful? Do pass on your tips to other sufferers and professionals. By sharing what is possible, it will enable and equip others to make their own recovery.

If you want to, you can share, your recovery journey and any additional tips with me, by email: thefatiguebook@gmail.com. I would be honoured to hear from you.

Let us all continue to share our knowledge and learning with one another. By doing this, the fatigue will get put in its place and people will not be alone on their road to recovery.

A society grows great when old men plant trees whose shade they know they shall never sit in.
Greek proverb

FOOD FOR THOUGHT

Life is an opportunity; benefit from it.

Life is a beauty; admire it.

Life is bliss; taste it.

Life is a dream; realise it.

Life is a challenge; meet it.

Life is a duty; complete it.

Life is a game; play it.

Life is costly; care for it.

Life is wealth; keep it.

Life is love; enjoy it.

Life is mystery; know it.

Life is a promise; fulfil it.

Life is a sorrow; overcome it.

Life is a song; sing it.

Life is a struggle; accept it.

Life is a tragedy; confront it.

Life is an adventure; dare it.

Life is luck; make it.

Life is too precious; do not destroy it.

Life is life; fight for it.[43]

Mother Teresa

PAUSE: MAKE SOME BROWNIES

You may have read this page title and thought that I had lost the plot. I assure you that I have not.

I started making brownies about 20 years ago, shortly after I was diagnosed with CFS/ME. Much of my world came to a stop and I was struggling. I was offered no help and, when I asked the doctor about the crippling cognitive difficulties that I was experiencing, I was told to try memorising telephone numbers from a directory. I cried and I have to confess that I never did follow that particular piece of advice.

I am incredibly thankful that I can now say that is an old narrative and that, after a lot of blood, sweat, tears, time and grace, my life and health are now in a very different place.

Back then, I discovered that making brownies was an easy and satisfying activity.

- I could make them over several days, if necessary: measure out the ingredients one day, cook them the next, chop them the next, share them the day after or freeze them for future days.

- I could stand up or sit down when preparing them.

- If they overcooked, they could be served with ice cream. If undercooked, they could be served half-frozen.

- They were an easy gift to make.

- They have marked many life events: births, marriages, deaths, as well as family and community celebrations. Somehow, they now have a life and reputation of their own.

Brownies may not be your thing – but something else might be.

I did not think they were 'my thing' but they have brought countless pleasures to many people over the years and that warms my heart. (See Brownie recipe, Appendix 5.)

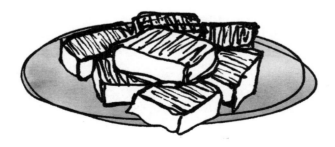

MIND, BODY AND SOUL: MAINTAIN PROGRESS – YOUR FUTURE

Mind: What were your thoughts as you read this chapter on Maintaining progress – your future?

Other parts of the chapter you can let go of for now.

Body: What actions will you start putting into practice?

Soul: You may want to seek soul help with these changes. As explained in the book's Introduction, this section is from my perspective as a Christian, inviting God's help in the recovery process. You may have your own way of seeking soul help, so please do what you feel comfortable with.

Dear God, I ask you for help with maintaining progress,
my future and my recovery journey.
'The LORD bless you and keep you;
'The LORD make his face shine on you and be gracious to you;
'The LORD turn his face towards you and give you peace.'^{NIV}
Thank you God
Amen – may it be so.
Based upon Numbers 6⁴⁴

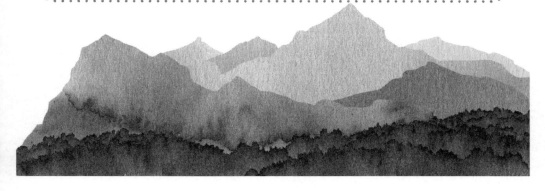

APPENDICES

APPENDIX 1 – ACTIVITY DIARY: HOW TO USE IT

Everything that you do in a day takes physical, mental or emotional energy. Getting out of bed, washing, dressing, eating, reading messages on your phone, climbing the stairs, talking to a family member, planning a shopping list, responding to an email, watching TV, etc. Write in hourly slots the main activity you were doing in that hour. Try to fill it in on a daily basis. Highlight or colour code the:

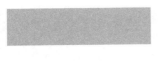 *Low-energy activities* – These activities require low energy. They are manageable and you hardly have to think about them. They have minimal after effects.

 *Medium-energy activities* – These activities require medium energy and are neither Low nor High.

 *High-energy activities* – These activities require a lot of energy. You would be unable to keep on performing them for extended periods of time. You may experience a certain amount of post-exertional malaise.

This is a subjective measure of what you consider to be low, medium or high-energy activities. This may vary from day to day depending upon how you are and the situation. At the end of each day, score your fatigue levels for that day between 0 and 10, where 0 = no fatigue and 10 = maximum fatigue.

I recommend doing this thoroughly for two weeks, then repeating it two months later and comparing the difference. Choose your own rhythm and what works for you but do not do it continuously.

After completing two weeks of activity diary sheets, ask yourself the following questions:

- What do I notice? What does that tell me?
- Where are the boom and bust patterns?
- Do the patterns correlate with high, medium, low-energy activities and the fatigue scores?
- Do my days and activities look quite balanced? If so, what did I do well? If not, what could I have done differently?
- How can I change next week's activities to be more balanced and spaced out?

- Have you made any other observations?

The following two Activity diary examples are based on a parent, with teenage children, who is on a phased return to part-time work (currently 14 hours a week).

These examples are for illustrative purposes only. Your Activity diary will be very different.

APPENDIX 1A – ACTIVITY DIARY: EXAMPLE OF BOOM AND BUST

Time	Monday	Tuesday	Wednesday
06.00-07.00	Sleep	Sleep	Sleep
07.00-08.00	Sleep	Sleep	Sleep
08.00-09.00	School Run	School Run	School Run
09.00-10.00	Back to Bed	Back to Bed	Medical Appointment
10.00-11.00	Sleep	Sleep	Medical Appointment
11.00-12.00	Wake up /Coffee	Wake up /Coffee	See Friend
12.00-13.00	Brunch	Brunch	Travel home
13.00-14.00	Work (from home)	Work (from home)	Work (from home)
14.00-15.00	Work (from home)	Work (from home)	Work (from home)
15.00-16.00	Work (from home)	Work (from home)	Headache lie on settee
16.00-17.00	Work (from home)	Work (from home)	Headache lie on settee
17.00-18.00	Meal prep & TV	Meal prep & TV	Order Take Away food
18.00-19.00	Meal with family	Meal with family	Meal with family
19.00-20.00	TV	TV	Argument
20.00-21.00	TV & nap	TV & nap	TV
21.00-22.00	TV	TV	TV
22.00-23.00	Bed – awake	Bed – awake	Bed – awake in pain
23.00-24.00	Bed – asleep	Bed – asleep	Bed – awake
Fatigue Score 1-10	10/10	10/10	10/10

Week commencing:

Thursday	Friday	Saturday	Sunday
Sleep	Bed – awake	Sleep	Sleep
Sleep	Sleep	Sleep	Sleep
Delegate School Run	Bed - awake	Bed - awake	Sleep
Back to Bed	Not Well	Bed - awake	Sleep
Not Well	Not Well	Laundry	Sleep
Not Well	Not Well	Look at Magazine	Get ready
Not Well	Phone Calls	Online Shopping	Out for meal with family
Not Well	Not Well	Listen to radio	Out for meal with family
Not Well	Not Well	Play short game	Out for meal with family
Not Well	TV	Preventative rest	Short walk
Not Well	Admin	Very short walk	Friend visited
Not Well	TV	TV	Nap
Take-Away meal for family	Meal with family	Left over's meal	Help with homework
Bed – early	TV	Few jobs	Snack with family
Bed - awake	Bath - Relax	TV	Bed - awake
Bed - awake	Bed - awake	Bath - Relax	Bed – awake
Bed - awake	Sleep	Bed - awake	Bed – awake
Sleep	Sleep	Sleep	Bed – awake
7/10	6/10	6/10	10/10

APPENDIX 1B – ACTIVITY DIARY: EXAMPLE OF PACING

Time	Monday	Tuesday	Wednesday
06.00-07.00	Sleep	Sleep	Sleep
07.00-08.00	Get ready/ Time on own	Get ready/ Time on own	Get ready/ Time on own
08.00-09.00	School Run	School Run	School Run
09.00-10.00	Breakfast/ Prev. Rest	Breakfast/ Prev. Rest	Breakfast/ Prev. Rest
10.00-11.00	Work 45m Prev. Rest 15m	Work 45m Prev. Rest 15m	Work 45m Prev. Rest 15m
11.00-12.00	Work 45m Prev. Rest 15m	Work 45m Prev. Rest 15m	Work 45m Prev. Rest 15m
12.00-13.00	Work 30m Lunch outside	Work 30m Lunch outside	Work 30m Lunch outside
13.00-14.00	Work 45m Prev. Rest 15m	Household jobs Prev. Rest	Work 45m Prev. Rest 15m
14.00-15.00	Work 30m Pilates 30m	Chat to friend Prev. Rest	Work 30m Pilates 30m
15.00-16.00	Work 45m Prev. Rest 15m	Knitting & TV	Work 45m Prev. Rest 15m
16.00-17.00	Meal prep/Short walk	Meal prep/Short walk	Meal prep/Short walk
17.00-18.00	TV	TV	TV
18.00-19.00	Meal with family	Meal with family	Meal with family
19.00-20.00	Knitting & TV	Pilates	Manicure & Music
20.00-21.00	TV	Help with Homework	TV
21.00-22.00	Bath/Relax in Bed	Bath/Relax in Bed	Bath/Relax in Bed
22.00-23.00	Sleep	Sleep	Sleep
23.00-24.00	Sleep	Sleep	Sleep
Fatigue Score	8/10	8/10	8/10

Week commencing:

Time	Thursday	Friday	Saturday	Sunday
06.00-07.00	Sleep	Sleep	Sleep	Sleep
07.00-08.00	Get ready/ Time on own	Get ready/ Time on own	Awake/ Relaxing	Awake/Relaxing
08.00-09.00	School Run	School Run	Get ready/ Time as couple	Get ready/ Time as couple
09.00-10.00	Breakfast/Prev. Rest	Breakfast/ Prev. Rest	Breakfast/ Prev. Rest	Breakfast/ Prev. Rest
10.00-11.00	Laundry	Work 45m / Prev. Rest 15m	Look at magazines	Jigsaw
11.00-12.00	TV	Work 45m / Prev. Rest 15m	Food delivery	Plan week / Prev. Rest
12.00-13.00	Phone call / Lunch outside	Work 30m / Lunch outside	Listen to radio	Family walk &
13.00-14.00	Pilates	Work 45m / Prev. Rest 15m	Family cleaning / Prev. Rest 15m	Prev. Rest / packed lunch
14.00-15.00	Online food shop	Work 30m / Pilates	Family cleaning / Prev. Rest 15m	TV
15.00-16.00	Sit in the garden	Work 45m / Prev. Rest 15m	Knitting & TV	Relative visit
16.00-17.00	Meal prep/Short walk	Meal prep/ Short walk	Short walk	Pilates
17.00-18.00	TV	TV	TV	TV
18.00-19.00	Meal with family	Meal with family	Ready Meal with family	Easy Meal with family
19.00-20.00	TV	Pedicure & Music	Pilates	Bit of tidying
20.00-21.00	Help with Homework	TV	Laundry	TV
21.00-22.00	Bath/Relax in Bed	Bath\Relax in Bed	Bath/Relax in Bed	Bath/Relax in Bed
22.00-23.00	Sleep	Sleep	Sleep	Sleep
23.00-24.00	Sleep	Sleep	Sleep	Sleep
Fatigue Score	6/10	8/10	7/10	7/10

APPENDIX 1C – ACTIVITY DIARY: FOR PHOTOCOPYING

Time	Monday	Tuesday	Wednesday
06.00-07.00			
07.00-08.00			
08.00-09.00			
09.00-10.00			
10.00-11.00			
11.00-12.00			
12.00-13.00			
13.00-14.00			
14.00-15.00			
15.00-16.00			
16.00-17.00			
17.00-18.00			
18.00-19.00			
19.00-20.00			
20.00-21.00			
21.00-22.00			
22.00-23.00			
23.00-24.00			
Fatigue Score			

Week commencing:

Thursday	Friday	Saturday	Sunday

APPENDIX 2 – REFLECTIVE SLEEP DIARY

What was I doing an hour before bedtime?

. . . .

How was I feeling in the evening? (Mark a cross on the line)

Sleepy •————————————————•————————————————• Alert

Relaxed •————————————————•————————————————• Tense

Happy •————————————————•————————————————• Sad

No Pain •————————————————•————————————————• Pain

What time did I get into bed?. . . . .
How long did it take me to fall asleep? Why? Any reasons?

. . . .

. . . .

Did I wake in the night? How often? Why? Any reasons?

. . . .

What time did I wake up?

. . . .

What time did I get up?

. . . .

How did I feel?

. . . .

How would I rate my night's sleep out of 10? (10 being excellent)

◄——►

0. . . . . **10**

I would recommend only doing this for a week or two, no more than that. That is enough time to recognise any patterns of sleep and highlight any particular areas that need concentrating on. Follow the tips in Chapter 3.

After completing a sleep diary for a few days answer the following statement:

If I could change the following, my sleep would improve:

1 . . . .

. . . .

2 . . . .

. . . .

3 . . . .

. . . .

APPENDIX 3 – PACING GROUP GUIDELINES

The aim of meeting in a small group, either in person or online, is to help support each other on your journey to recovery. This is not a social time nor a time to hear in detail how each person is. Those conversations can be held at another time, perhaps on a WhatsApp group or something similar. Having clear and precise guidelines enables the group to model pacing – thus you can care for your own needs whilst benefiting from social interaction and peer support.

The frequency of meeting – Ideally once a fortnight.

The time of the meeting is at a prearranged time of the day that is suitable for all members. As far as you are able, be punctual and stick to the schedule.

The size of the group should be no more than three people.

The roles of each person:

- Person 1 to be the precise timekeeper. If people run over, the whole group will experience too much fatigue. It is really important to keep to time

- Person 2 to read out the questions and facilitate each person taking turns

- Person 3 to clarify the date and time of the next meeting and send out Zoom links or practical details

The equipment:

- Each person has a copy of *The Fatigue Book*.

- A 'Time out' card of any colour. You show the card to indicate you are taking an additional break, as and when you may need to. Using the card does not interrupt the meeting or expect an explanation. In your absence other group members can take on your role.

- Notebook and pen.

The preparation – Spend some time the day before looking at the discussion questions and writing down your thoughts. Preparing the day before allows you to pace your cognitive energy.

The schedule – plan to meet for no longer than 60 minutes.

First meeting guidelines

Greetings (0.00 – 0.05 (5 minutes))

- Decide who is Person 1, 2 and 3.

- Person 3 arranges and confirms the date and time for the next meeting.

- Person 3 then hands over to Person 2.

Discussion 1 (0.05 – 0.20 (15 minutes)) Person 2 facilitates.

- What do you hope to gain from the group meetings?

- What do you hope to contribute to the group meetings?

Break (0.20 – 0.25 (5 minutes))

Stand up if you are able – move away from the computer, stretch, be quiet and do not talk. Person 1 calls everyone back after 5 minutes.

Discussion 2 (0.25 – 0.40 (15 minutes)) Person 2 facilitates.

- What may help you in benefitting from time together?

- What may hinder you in benefitting from time together?

Break (0.40 – 0.45 (5 minutes))

Stand up if you are able – move away from the computer, stretch, be quiet and do not talk. Person 1 calls everyone back after 5 minutes.

Discussion 3 (0.45 – 1.00 (15 minutes)) Person 2 facilitates.

- Share one of your own tips that has helped you in your journey so far.

Meeting closed

In preparation for the second meeting:
- Read Chapter 1 – Your story early this week.

- The day before the planned meeting, spend some time looking at the discussion questions and writing down your thoughts.

Regular fortnightly meeting guidelines

Greetings (0.00 – 0.05 (5 minutes))

- Decide who is Person 1, 2 and 3.
- Person 3 arranges and confirms the date and time for the next meeting.
- Person 3 then hands over to Person 2.

Discussion 1 (0.05 – 0.20 (15 minutes)) Person 2 facilitates.

- What was your main take-away tip from this chapter and why?
- If there is time, discuss other tips.

Break (0.20 – 0.25 (5 minutes))

Stand up if you are able – move away from the computer, stretch, be quiet and do not talk. Person 1 calls everyone back after 5 minutes.

Discussion 2 (0.25 – 0.40 (15 minutes)) Person 2 facilitates.

- What changes have you made as a result of this chapter?

Break (0.40 – 0.45 (5 minutes))

Stand up if you are able – move away from the computer, stretch, be quiet and do not talk. Person 1 calls everyone back after 5 minutes.

Discussion 3 (0.45 – 1.00 (15 minutes)) Person 2 facilitates

- How do you plan to continue applying this in the coming weeks?
- What may help and what may hinder?

Clarify which chapter to discuss at the next meeting. You may choose to stay with this chapter or continue with the next.

Meeting closed

In preparation for the subsequent meetings:
- Read or re-read the chapter early in the week.
- The day before the planned meeting, spend some time looking at the discussion questions and writing down your thoughts.

APPENDIX 4 – WHEEL OF LIFE: BLANK FOR PHOTOCOPYING

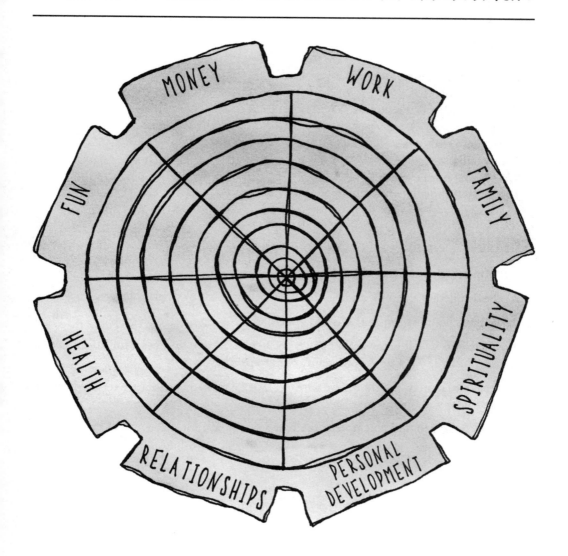

APPENDIX 5 – BROWNIE RECIPE

INGREDIENTS

225 g (8oz) granulated sugar
50 g (2oz) cocoa
75 g (3oz) self-raising flour
½ tsp salt
2 medium sized eggs
2 tbsp milk
125 g (5oz) butter, melted
100 g (4oz) chocolate bar, chopped into small pieces

METHOD

1. Mix together the dry ingredients.

2. Beat together the milk and eggs and add along with the melted butter.

3. Mix well and stir in the chopped chocolate.

4. Pour into a well-greased tin (9"x 9"/ 23 cm x 23 cm) and bake for 20-30 minutes at 180°C/350°F/Gas 4 until gently firm to touch.

5. Leave to cool in the tin before cutting. Drizzle melted chocolate over the brownies and dust with icing sugar.

6. Can be frozen and will store in a tin in a cool place for up to a week.

ACKNOWLEDGEMENTS

In closing I would like to thank the many people who have co-created this book. You know who you are. I could not have done this without each and every one of you. Your support and contribution has shaped what this book has become.

I am forever grateful.

Mostly, I thank the countless people I have worked with over the years. Those of you, who have journeyed with the ups and downs of the chronic fatigue. Sharing parts of your story with me changed my outlook and taught me all I know.

I am forever grateful.

Finally I thank you the reader for picking up this book in the first place. May it provide you with some hope for your journey ahead – Go well.

I am forever grateful.

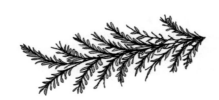

REFERENCES

1. Office For National Statistics (ONS). Prevalence of ongoing symptoms following coronavirus (COVID-19) infection in the UK. 2021. Available from: www.ons.gov.uk/peoplepopulationandcommunity/healthandsocialcare/conditionsanddiseases/bulletins/prevalenceofongoingsymptomsfollowingcoronaviruscovid19infectionintheuk/1april2021 [Accessed 4 January 2022]

2. Office For National Statistics (ONS). Prevalence of ongoing symptoms following coronavirus (COVID-19) infection in the UK. 2022. Available from: www.ons.gov.uk/peoplepopulationandcommunity/healthandsocialcare/conditionsanddiseases/bulletins/prevalenceofongoingsymptomsfollowingcoronaviruscovid19infectionintheuk/7april2022 [Accessed 21 April 2022]

3. National Institute for Health and Care Excellence (NICE). COVID-19 rapid guideline: managing the long-term effects of COVID-19: NICE Guideline (NG188). 2020, last updated 2021. Available from: www.nice.org.uk/guidance /ng188/chapter/Recommendations [Accessed 19 January 2022]

4. National Institute for Health and Care Excellence (NICE), Myalgic encephalomyelitis (or encephalopathy)/chronic fatigue syndrome: diagnosis and management : NICE Guideline[NG206]. 2021. Available from: www.nice.org.uk/guidance/ng206 (Accessed 19 January 2022)

5. Shakespeare W. *Romeo & Juliet*. Act II, Scene III. Available from: www.opensourceshakespeare.org/views/plays/play_view.php?WorkID=romeojuliet&Act=2&Scene=3&Scope=scene [Accessed 3 April 2022]

6. *The Holy Bible*. NIV. Grand Rapids, MI: Zondervan; 2011. Print. Psalm 139:10, 13-18.

7. National Institute for Health and Care Excellence (NICE), Myalgic encephalomyelitis(or encephalopathy) /chronic fatigue syndrome: diagnosis and management[G] Evidence reviews for the non-pharmacological management of ME/CFS NICE guideline NG206 Evidence reviews underpinning recommendations and research recommendations in the NICE guideline. 2021. Available from: www.nice.org.uk/guidance/ng206/evidence/g-nonpharmacological-management-of-mecfs-pdf-9265183028 [Accessed 3 February 2022]

8. Health and Safety Executive (UK). *Human factors: Fatigue and shift work - Why is fatigue important*. Available from: www.hse.gov.uk/humanfactors /topics/fatigue.htm [Accessed 20 January 2022]

9. Cuddy A. *Your Body Language May Shape Who You Are*. Houston: TEDx; 2012. Available from: www.ted.com/talks/amy_cuddy_your_body_ language_may_shape_who_you_are/transcript [Accessed 20 January 2022]

10. *The Holy Bible*. NIV. Grand Rapids, MI: Zondervan; 2011. Print. Matthew 11: 28-30.

11. Walker M. *Why We Sleep: Unlocking the Power of Sleep and Dreams*. New York, USA: Simon & Schuster, USA; 2017, p.340.

12. The Holy Bible. NIV. Grand Rapids, MI: Zondervan; 2011. Print. Psalm 121: 1-4, 8.

13. Clear J. *How Long Does it Actually Take to Form a New Habit? (Backed by Science)*. Available from: https://jamesclear.com/new-habit [Accessed 25 November 2021]

14. Fisher J. Process of Personal Transition. 2012. Available from the businessballs.com website: www.businessballs.com/change-management/personal-change-stages-john-fisher/ [Accessed 1 June 2021]

15. West R. Time for a change: Putting the Transtheoretical (Stages of Change) Model to rest [Editorial]. *Addiction 2005; 100*(8): 1036-1039. doi/10.1111/j.1360-0443.2005. 01139.x [Accessed 25 January 2022]

16. Newman L. Elisabeth Kübler-Ross. *BMJ* 2004; 329(7466): 627.

17. Strong T, Pyle, NR. Constructing a conversational "miracle": Examining the "miracle question" as it is used in therapeutic dialogue. *Journal of Constructivist Psychology* 2009; 22(4): 328–353.

18. Mandela N. *Long Walk to Freedom*. London: Abacus; 2013 [1995].

19. The Holy Bible. NIV. Grand Rapids, MI: Zondervan; 2011. Print. Isaiah 42:16.

20. DENT Neurological Institute. *22 Facts About the Brain | World Brain Day*. Available from: www.dentinstitute.com/posts/lifestyle-tips/22-facts-about-the-brain-world-brain-day/ [Accessed 2 December 2021]

21. *The Holy Bible*. NIV. Grand Rapids, MI: Zondervan; 2011. Print. Isaiah 40:31.

22. *Bateson G. Steps to an Ecology of Mind: Collected Essays in Anthropology, Psychiatry, Evolution, and Epistemology. Chicago: University of Chicago Press; 2000 [1972], p 453.*

23. *The Holy Bible*. NIV. Grand Rapids, MI: Zondervan; 2011. Print. Proverbs 3: 5-8.

24. ten Boom C. *Clippings From My Notebook*. London, Great Britain: Triangle, SPCK; 1994 [1982], p 20.

25. Bergland C. Diaphragmatic Breathing Exercises and your Vagus Nerve. Psychology Today. Available from: www.psychologytoday.com/gb/blog/the-athletes-way/201705/diaphragmatic-breathing-exercises-and-your-vagus-nerve [Accessed 25th January 2022]

26. *The Holy Bible*. NIV. Grand Rapids, MI: Zondervan; 2011. Print. 1 Peter 5:7, Philippians 4:6-7.

27. Carers UK. *State of Caring - A snapshot of unpaid care in the UK- 2019*. Available from: www.carersuk.org/images/News__campaigns /CUK_State_of_Caring_2019_Report.pdf [Accessed 1 February 2022]

28. British Heart Foundation. *Sex when you have a heart or circulatory condition - your questions answered*. Available from: www.bhf.org.uk/ informationsupport/heart-matters-magazine/wellbeing/sex-when-you-have-a-heart-condition/faqs-about-sex-and-heart-disease [Accessed 23 January 2022]

29. James W. *The Letters of William James, Vol. II*. Urbana, Illinois: Project Gutenberg; 2011. Available from: www.gutenberg.org/ebooks/38091. [Accessed 10 March 2022]

30. Brown B. *The Gifts of Imperfection*. Minnesota, USA: Hazelden, USA; 2010, p.19.

31. *The Holy Bible*. NIV. Grand Rapids, MI: Zondervan; 2011. Print. 1 Corinthians 13: 4-8.

32. Mukamal R, American Academy of Ophthalmology. *All About Emotional Tears*. Available from: www.aao.org/eye-health/tips-prevention/all-about-emotional-tears [Accessed 3 February 2022]

33. Brabban A, Turkington D. The search for meaning: Detecting congruence between life events, underlying schema and psychotic symptoms. In: Morrison AP. (ed.) *A Casebook of cognitive therapy for psychosis*. East Sussex: Brunner, Routledge; 2002, p. 59-77.

34. Wikipedia: the free encyclopedia. Kitsugi. Available from: https://en.wikipedia.org/wiki/Kintsugi [Accessed 2 January 2022]

35. BBC News. NHS could give therapy before anti-depressants, under new guidelines. 2021. Available from: www.bbc.co.uk/news/ health-59383722 [Accessed 1 December 2021]

36. National Institute for Health and Care Excellence (NICE), NICE creates new menu of treatment options for those suffering from depression: NICE. 2021. Available from: www.nice.org.uk/news/nice-creates-new-menu-of-treatment-options-for-those-suffering-from-depression [Accessed 2 February 2022]

37. English National Opera. *About the ENO Breathe Programme*. Available from: www.eno.org/eno-breathe/about-the-eno-breathe-programme/ [Accessed 3 February 2022]

38. Ackerman CE. Positive Psychology.com. *How Does Acceptance And Commitment Therapy (ACT) Work?* Available from: https://positivepsychology.com/act-acceptance-and-commitment-therapy/ [Accessed 3 December 2021]

39. Wikipedia: the free encyclopedia. Serenity Prayer; Available from: https://en.wikipedia.org/wiki/Serenity_Prayer [Accessed 2 February 2022]

40. Davis HE, Assaf GS, McCorkell L, Wei H, Low RJ, Re'em Y, et al. Characterizing long COVID in an International Cohort: 7 Months of Symptoms and Their Impact. *eClinical Medicine* 2021; 38: 101019. doi.org/10.1016/j.eclinm.2021.101019

41. *The Holy Bible*. NIV. Grand Rapids, MI: Zondervan; 2011. Print. Isaiah 41:10,13-14.

42. Holman HR. The Relation of the Chronic Disease Epidemic to the Health Care Crisis. *ACR Open Rheumatol* 2020; 2(3): 167-173. doi.org/10.1002/acr2.11114

43. U.O.F. *Mother Teresa - Life Is*. Available from: https://universeoffaith.org/life-is-a-poem-by-mother-teresa/ [Accessed 3 November 2021]

44. *The Holy Bible*. NIV. Grand Rapids, MI: Zondervan; 2011. Print. Numbers 6:24-26.

100 TIPS

INDEX

ENDORSEMENTS

I could not be happier than to recommend this guide for those grappling with the far-reaching effects of long COVID and chronic fatigue. This book will be equally beneficial to those personally affected by fatigue, their families and friends and to the professionals involved in their care. Lydia's wealth of clinical experience, her understanding and wisdom, and her ability to communicate all of this knowledge in such a compassionate and constructive way are a rare combination. Her warmth and gentle curiosity emanate from the pages of this book. Dr Theresa Wynne, Clinical Psychologist

This delightfully illustrated book combines compassion, experience and insight. For those wearied by the constant battle with fatigue, this book offers an accessible, digestible and oh-so-beautifully-put- together travelling partner into a journey of constructive change. I wholeheartedly and highly recommend this book for those seeking to find a way through the weightiness of fatigue in a gentle, strategically paced and personally meaningful way. Suzanne Elizabeth Davis, Physiotherapist and Family Therapist

Lydia's book offers gentle, nurtured guidance on how to manage the experience of chronic fatigue. Her voice is compassionate and wise, where the wealth of her experience jumps off the page. She provides practical, achievable tips to improve wellbeing and offers encouragement and positivity throughout. I have learnt even more from reading it and can fully endorse the transformative effect that implementing her ideas will have. Savour every word of this precious gift! Linzi Bound, Occupational Therapist and Mindfulness Teacher

I particularly like the warm conversational tone, the consistent message of positivity, hope and realistic expectation of progress. With its wide range of topics, it strikes me as a book people could dip in and out of, depending upon what particular difficulties they want to focus on. I love the illustrations; they really support the text and make it more visually engaging and less daunting than the solid text; the highlighted sections help people focus on key messages so they don't feel overwhelmed. Dr Jayne Woodcock, Clinical Psychologist